# YOGA FOR PREGNANCY

*Safe and Gentle Stretches*

# YOGA FOR
# PREGNANCY

*Safe and Gentle Stretches*

by Sandra Jordan

St. Martin's Press
New York

*Design by Allen Hicks and Rowen Tabusa*

Library of Congress Cataloging-in-Publication Data

Jordan, Sandra.
  Yoga for pregnancy / Sandra Jordan.
    p.    cm.
  ISBN 0-312-02322-7
  1. Pregnancy.  2. Exercise for women.  3. Yoga, Hatha.
I. Title.
RG558.7.J67  1988
618.2'4—dc19                      88-16887
                                              CIP

Originally published by Sun Moon, Inc., under the title *Yoga During Pregnancy*.

First Edition
20 19 18 17 16 15

**NOTE TO THE READER**:
Each individual is different, and no stretching or exercise program is ideal for every individual. Accordingly, the reader should consult with a physician before undertaking and while progressing through this or any other yoga or prenatal program. This is especially important if the reader has any medical condition or is taking any medication that might be affected by such a program. Neither this nor any other book should be used as a substitute for professional medical care or treatment.

*For Glenn*
*without whose love, friendship, advice, and hard work*
*this book would never have been completed*

*and for my sons Michael and Jeffrey*
*who bring me joy*

# Acknowledgments

I wish to acknowledge the following teachers with whom I have studied:

Mr. B. K. S. Iyengar for his profound knowledge of yoga freely shared through his teaching.

Geeta Iyengar for imparting her understanding of yoga for the special needs of women.

Judith Lasater for combining anatomy and intuition in the teaching of yoga.

Larry Hatlett for sharing his warmth and awareness of yoga.

Glenn Kawana for his perceptive approach to the teaching of yoga.

I appreciate Gloria Ascher's careful reading of the text and her thoughtful suggestions.

I am grateful to Sandra Penn, M.D. for reviewing the introductory chapter information and photographs.

I sincerely wish to thank the following women from my prenatal yoga classes who posed for these photos:

Jackie Barnes                    Karla Brom
Julia Cammarata-Straus           Susan Des Jarlais
Janet Doll-Scarfone              Robin Gruver
Kathy Jackson

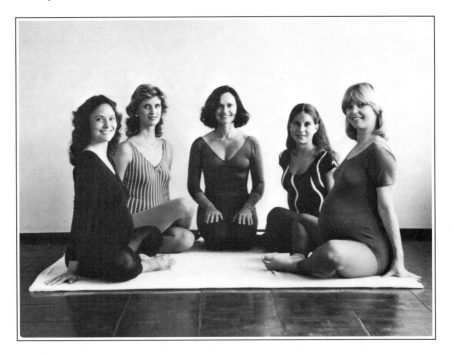

# Table Of Contents

# Foreword

One of my great pleasures has come from taking care of pregnant women, watching them grow along with their children. There are so many do's and don'ts these days, it is a wonder that so many women still approach pregnancy with enthusiasm! There are childbirth classes, and parenting classes, books, and videos. And this is in addition to the tremendous daily inundation from radio, television, newspapers and magazines.

I have referred my patients to Sandra's classes for the support she offers - the gentle, caring awareness of each pregnant woman's emerging motherhood, her changing body, and its potential for suppleness. And the delight of these women has been, not only for the control they discover, but also for the contemplative environment which they find so peaceful. Quiet mindfulness is rare and so needed when so much else is changing. It is a welcomed place for the wonder and mystery of growing life and giving birth.

This book provides an easy to follow guide to the postures of Iyengar yoga, with careful attention to their appropriateness for pregnancy. Sandra's trimester coding is clear. Her postures are chosen to avoid unhealthy stress in late pregnancy. The photographs, along with the concise descriptions, are elegant in their simplicity. It will be a welcomed companion for quiet, self expression.

Sandra F. Penn, M.D.
Family Practice

# YOGA FOR PREGNANCY

*Safe and Gentle Stretches*

# Introduction

Yoga is an ideal preparation for labor and birth. It is also an excellent way to get back into shape after birth. The reason for this lies in yoga's approach. To experience yoga you need to be fully involved. The attention of the mind and the awareness of the breath are added to the movements of the body.

The physical positions of yoga are called poses or postures, not exercises. The word exercise conveys a feeling of movement. The word pose expresses a feeling of moving into stillness. In yoga the body is eased into alignment with the awareness of the breath. The pose is then held quietly until the mind and the body are in tune.

Performing yoga poses with awareness creates a state of calmness. When a pregnant women feels inner clarity, her confidence grows. When she feels peaceful, her anxiety concerning the birth process decreases.

The mind becomes involved in the body movements. This focus allows the pregnant woman to tune out distracting forces around her during labor and to respond appropriately to the contractions.

I recently watched one of my pregnant students give birth, and I was impressed by her concentration. She told me as labor progressed she was able to adjust the way she handled the pushing contractions as the baby changed position. She was following the movements of the baby with her body, breath, and mind.

This ability to focus takes practice. Yoga provides a way to refine the movements of the body. When first performing the poses, you may feel slightly awkward and stiff. Continue to do the same poses, and perform them at any pace you choose. After practicing them over and over again, the body will stretch, adapt, and gradually move into alignment.

As you get to know your body through practicing yoga poses, you will be confronted with your physical strengths and weaknesses. This is invaluable training, for labor is a very physical process. Knowing where you are tight or weak, and working on those areas, will help you prepare your body for birth.

As you feel the growth of the baby within, you need also to experience your own inner growth. Therefore yoga is not a type of exercise to be learned. It is an approach to be understood. The yoga way is a calm, mindful way, not given to extremes. Experiment with the yoga poses not only as physical techniques to be acquired, but also as a mental and emotional preparation for birth.

This approach offers no guarantees for an easier or quicker birth. However, your increased body awareness and enhanced ability to breathe and relax will help you adjust to the physical demands of labor, birth, and motherhood.

# When To Begin Yoga During Pregnancy

Before beginning any prenatal exercise program, it is necessary to obtain your physician's consent. Certain conditions would make exercise uncomfortable or unsafe.

Do not exercise strenuously if you have a history of miscarriages, or cervical insufficiency. During pregnancy the cervix should remain tight to prevent infection.

It would be unsafe to exercise with a previous back injury such as a herniated disc.

In the first trimester of pregnancy, many women experience fatigue, nausea, and dizziness. It is best to wait until these conditions have subsided before beginning a program of exercise.

The yoga postures in this book have all been adapted to be safe for pregnant women. Each pose is clearly labeled. The number of suitable trimesters is indicated in the upper right hand corner of each pose description.

Yoga postures are used throughout this book because yoga is appropriate for pregnant women. The yoga poses stress a mindful, focused attitude toward practice. They have as their goals the creation of a balanced body and a calm mind.

# General Hints And Cautions

Observe the following hints and cautions when practicing yoga postures on your own. It is always best to learn under the guidance of a qualified teacher. However, with these cautions in mind, doing the poses can be safe, effective, and enjoyable.

☐ Practice in a cool, quiet, and well-ventilated room. Place blankets, pillows, a folding chair, and mat or rug nearby.

☐ Wear loose, comfortable clothing which will not restrict movement. Do all the poses with bare feet.

☐ Practice poses for 15 to 20 minutes a day. Allow 5 to 10 minutes for breathing and relaxation. If time permits, you may gradually increase the total time to one hour.

- ☐ Perform the standing poses with one heel to the wall, or use a chair for support. Place hands on the wall for support and balance.

- ☐ Preserve the normal curves of the spine. When bending forward, bend from the hips, not the back. Maintain as much distance as possible between the breastbone and the pubic bone. Keeping the back straight will make breathing easier.

- ☐ Avoid poses which overstretch the abdominal muscles. Keep the pelvis upright when stretching the chest and the front of the thighs. The upright pelvis and lifted spine will improve posture.

- ☐ When bending forward in a sitting position, place a strap around the feet, hold the strap with both hands, bend from the hips, and lift the chest. The erect position of the spine will prevent lower back strain and compression of the abdomen.

- ☐ When practicing twisting poses, turn without putting any pressure on the abdomen. Concentrate the twist mainly in the shoulder, rib cage, and upper back areas.

- ☐ After the fourth month discontinue all back-lying poses. Practice breathing sitting with the back to the wall, and relax in a side-lying position.

- ☐ Listen carefully to your body. Each month you will need to adapt to the changes occuring within you. Cease practicing a pose whenever it no longer feels good.

# How To Use This Book

This book includes photos and descriptions of 78 prenatal yoga poses and 14 postnatal yoga poses. Each page contains a symbol, in the upper right hand corner, indicating the number of trimesters suitable for the practice of the pose. The explanation of the four symbols is as follows:

### Poses Suitable For The First Trimester Of Pregnancy
Many of the poses with the first trimester symbol include back-lying positions which should be discontinued after the fourth month.

### Poses Suitable For The First And Second Trimesters Of Pregnancy
The poses for first and second trimesters emphasize standing poses for strength and balance, and sitting poses for flexibility. They may be too vigorous for the third trimester.

### Poses Suitable For The First, Second, And Third Trimesters Of Pregnancy
All poses with this symbol may be practiced safely during the entire pregnancy. Poses using a chair for support are ideal for the third trimester.

### Poses Suitable For The Postpartum Period Following Childbirth
The poses with the postnatal symbol emphasize abdominal strengthening, twisting, and relaxation. Poses from the prenatal sections may also be included.

# How To Organize A Program Of Yoga Poses

The poses in the first eight chapters are grouped by areas of the body. You may decide to create a balanced practice session by performing one pose from each chapter. Or you may do appropriate poses from just one or two sections. For example, if the backs of your legs feel tight, you might do hamstring stretching postures from Chapter 6 combined with standing poses from Chapter 3.

Chapter 9 offers a complete postnatal program. Or if your shoulders are tight from nursing and carrying the baby, you may do shoulder stretching poses from Chapter 2.

At the end of Chapter 9 there are three sample yoga programs. Each program of 12 poses is suitable for one of the three trimesters of pregnancy.

To make practicing yoga even more enjoyable, include a daily time for deep breathing and relaxation.

# Chapter 1

# THE PELVIC TILTING POSES

The proper positioning of the pelvis is the key to correct posture. The placement of the pelvis determines the curves of the spine. When the pelvis is correctly placed, the supporting structures above it will move into balance. All in all it is an *awareness* of good posture which will bring the whole body into alignment.

A normal back has four curves. They form an **S** shape. The lower back and neck are *concave curves* - they curve inward toward the front of the body. The tailbone area and the upper back are *convex curves* - they curve outward away from the back of the body.

The normal curves of the back insure proper spacing between the vertebrae of the back. Nerves branch out from the spinal cord and exit between the vertebrae. If the curves become excessive or flattened, compression of the nerves which pass between the vertebrae may result.

Pregnancy tends to cause compression in the lower back. This compression is due to the weight of the growing uterus and the subsequent lack of abdominal muscle control. As a result, correct posture is distorted. This creates an excessive lower back curve. Reclining pelvic tilting poses will help alleviate this compression. The accompanying lower back pain will be relieved by lengthening the lower back muscles.

Pelvic tilting on hands and knees (Cat Stretch p. 4) may also relieve back pain and sciatica. The emphasis is on working the abdominal muscles against gravity. This hands and knees position may also be used in labor to relieve backache.

# Hints And Cautions

Pelvic tilting poses may be performed during all three trimesters of pregnancy. However back-lying pelvic tilts should be limited to the first trimester.

After the fourth or fifth month a pregnant woman lying on her back may become uncomfortable, dizzy, or even nauseous. This is due to the weight of the uterus pressing down on a vein called the vena cava. The vena cava brings blood back to the heart from the legs and pelvis. When it is compressed, blood volume to the heart decreases, blood pressure drops, and blood flow to the mother's brain and the placenta is lessened. This causes temporary oxygen deprivation to mother and child. If this should happen, the mother would become light-headed. To stop the dizziness, she would need to roll onto her side and sit up.

The *vena cava syndrome* is most pronounced in the last trimester of pregnancy. Therefore, all back-lying poses are to be discontinued after the fifth month.

It is important to prevent straining the abdominal muscles during pregnancy. They are already being over-stretched by the growing uterus. To avoid overworking these muscles when sitting up, roll onto one side, and use your hands to push yourself up to a sitting position.

# Basic Standing Posture

- [ ] Stand erect with feet slightly apart and outer edges of feet parallel to each other. Distribute weight of body evenly over arches of feet.

- [ ] Completely straighten legs by tightening front thigh muscles.

- [ ] To create horizontal alignment of pelvis, lift up front hipbones and move tailbone down toward floor.

- [ ] Lift breastbone up and slightly forward. Drop shoulders and relax arms. Lengthen back of neck and look directly forward. Ankles, hips, shoulders, and ears should be in line. Adjust standing position as pregnancy progresses.

- [ ] Standing correctly improves posture and relieves lower back strain by balancing muscles and aligning vertebrae.

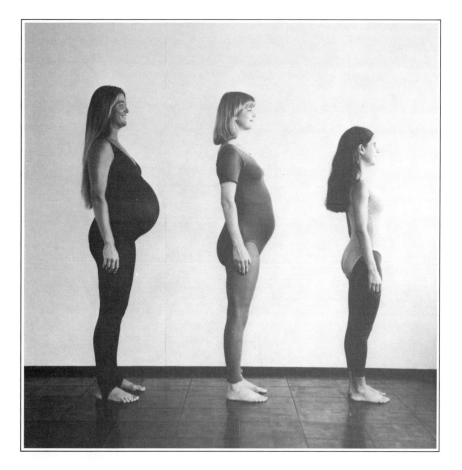

# Reclining Pelvic Tilt

☐ Lie on back on mat. Bend knees and place feet flat on mat. Feet are apart, parallel, and a comfortable distance from buttocks. Knees may relax inward until they touch. Extend arms at sides with palms facing upward.

☐ Breathe in, lift chest, and allow lower back to arch and lift slightly off floor.

☐ Breathe out, press feet firmly, and flatten lower back to floor. Tighten buttock muscles and let tailbone lift slightly off of floor.

☐ Repeat pelvic tilt 5 to 10 times. Inhale and release lower back, exhale and press lower back to lengthen spinal muscles. When finished roll onto one side and sit up.

☐ This pose relieves tension in lower back muscles.

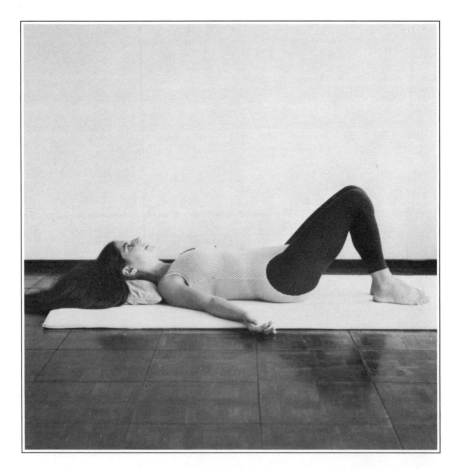

# Bridge Pose

☐ Lie on back, bend knees, and place feet flat on mat. Feet are apart, parallel, and a comfortable distance from buttocks. With palms down, stretch arms alongside body.

☐ Exhale, press lower back firmly to floor. Inhale and tighten buttocks. On next exhalation, press down with arms and feet, lift hips off floor, and raise tailbone upward. Lengthen lower back while lifting. Breathe normally and hold. Roll down and relax.

☐ Repeat 2 or 3 times. Curl tailbone off floor first, lift pelvis higher than abdomen, and squeeze knees together. Release, gently lowering upper back to floor first. Roll onto one side and push up to a sitting position.

☐ This pose relieves lower back pain by strengthening abdominal and buttock muscles.

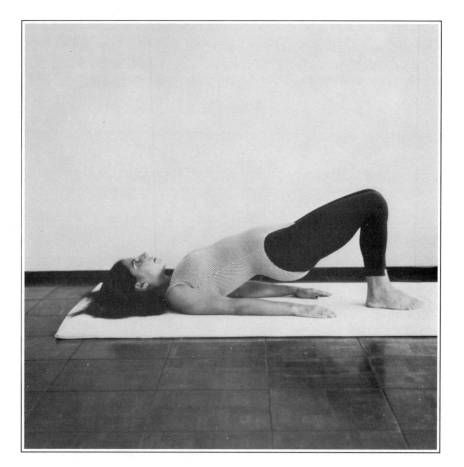

# Cat Stretch

☐ Kneel on floor. Position knees directly under hips and a few inches apart. Place hands in line with shoulders, fingers facing forward. Look straight ahead.

☐ While inhaling, look up, lift buttocks, and descend lower back slightly.

☐ While exhaling, look down, tuck buttocks under, lift back, and allow upper back to round upward.

☐ Repeat 5 times. Inhale and release back downward. Exhale and lift back upward. Keep arms straight. Release, sit back on heels, widen legs, stretch spine forward between legs, and rest forehead on floor.

☐ This pose releases lower back tension, and is excellent during back labor.

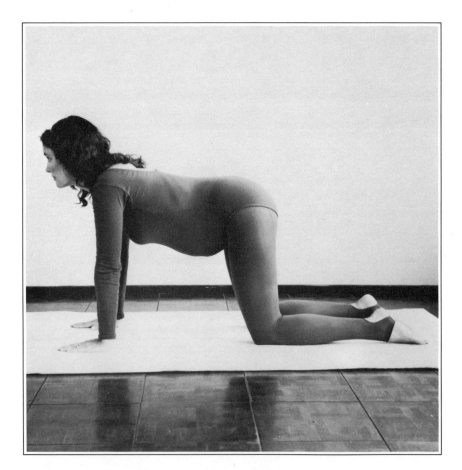

# Cat Stretch With Leg Lift

☐ Kneel on floor. Position knees directly under hips and a few inches apart. Place hands in line with shoulders, fingers facing forward.

☐ While inhaling, look up, lift buttocks, tilt top of front pelvis downward, and allow lower back to descend slightly. While exhaling, look down, tuck buttocks under, lift back, and allow upper back to round upward.

☐ Return to neutral position on hands and knees. Look forward and maintain natural spinal curves.

☐ Extend left leg on floor, turn toes under to stretch calf muscles. Lift leg off floor, hold, and alternately point and flex foot. Lower leg and repeat with right leg.

☐ This pose strengthens back, buttock, hamstring, calf and shin muscles.

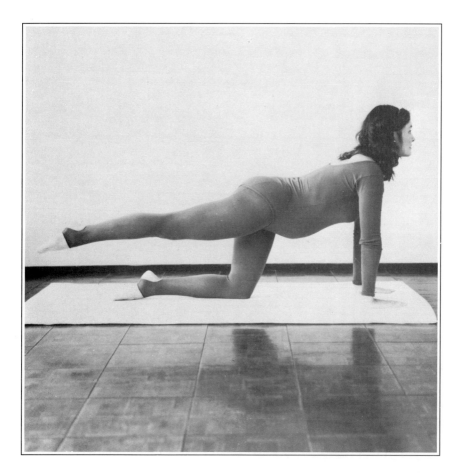

# Lower Back Stretch To Wall

☐ Stand with back to wall and position feet a few inches from wall. Separate feet, bend knees slightly, and rest hands on thighs. Feet are parallel to each other and knees face straight ahead.

☐ Inhale and lengthen spine. Exhale, tuck tailbone under, and flatten lower back to wall. Breathe normally and maintain stretch of lower back against wall.

☐ Use this resting pose frequently when back is tired. Hands may rest on wall, or interlock underneath abdomen, for support in last trimester. To strengthen thigh muscles, bend knees, lower buttocks until thighs are almost parallel to floor, and press lower back to wall.

☐ To release, straighten legs, and stand in upright position.

☐ This pose relieves lower back fatigue and strengthens legs.

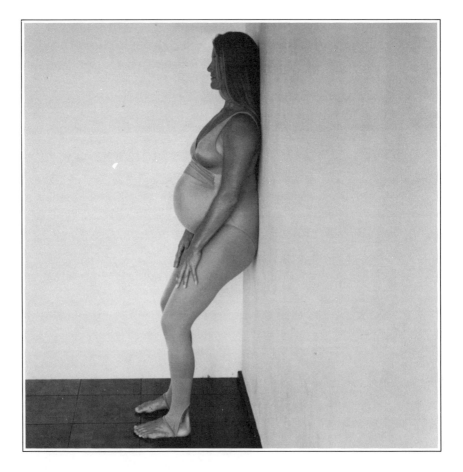

# Chapter 2

# THE SHOULDER STRETCHING AND CHEST OPENING POSES

Supple shoulders and a movable rib cage make free breathing in the chest possible. Tight chest, neck, and shoulder muscles create tension. Stretching may temporarily relieve this tightness. However, chronic shoulder tightness during pregnancy may be due to incorrect posture or not enough exercise. Poor posture may be corrected by strengthening weak upper back muscles, loosening stiff shoulders, and expanding the chest.

In poor posture the chest collapses, the shoulders round forward, and the upper back hunches over. These actions restrict the movement of the rib cage. As the pregnancy progresses, the space available for breathing becomes less and less. To breathe deeply, it is essential to allow the rib cage to expand.

The following shoulder stretches and chest opening poses will help correct faulty posture by strengthening the muscles which pull the shoulder blades down and together, and stretching the muscles of the rib cage. As the chest expands, the lungs gain freedom, and breathing deepens.

After the baby is born, these poses will help relieve shoulder tension caused by nursing and carrying the baby.

# Hints And Cautions

When doing shoulder stretches, be careful not to sway the lower back too much. Concentrate on lengthening the back.

If there is pain, weakness, or numbness in the wrists in the Downward Dog poses, you may have *carpal tunnel syndrome*. In this condition hormonal changes or weight gain cause fluid to accumulate in the wrists. This creates pressure on the median nerve in the wrist. Avoid poses which place downward pressure on the palms. This condition usually disappears after childbirth.

# Shoulder Stretch
# With Chair

- ☐ Place back of chair to wall. Kneel on mat or pillows. Separate knees a comfortable distance apart.

- ☐ Place elbows securely on chair seat and no farther apart than shoulder width. Lift forearms toward ceiling and press palms together. Allow neck to relax. If comfortable, head may drop between arms toward floor.

- ☐ Breathe normally. Relax shoulders and back. Tilt pelvis slightly and lift buttocks toward ceiling. With each exhalation descend chest and shoulders toward floor.

- ☐ To release, lower hands onto chair, push back, sit on heels, and relax arms alongside body.

- ☐ This pose stretches shoulders. Rest elbows on edge of bed during labor. This pose relieves pain of back labor.

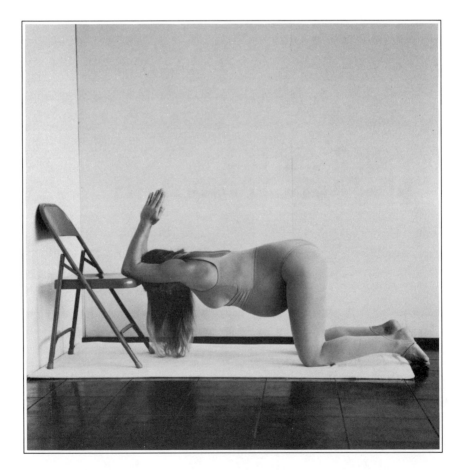

# Forearms On Wall
# Shoulder Stretch

☐ Interlock fingers, place forearms high up on wall, and walk feet back until legs are directly under hips.

☐ Place feet parallel to each other, tighten front thigh muscles, and release head between arms. Forehead may rest lightly on wall.

☐ Inhale and press forearms to wall. Exhale and descend shoulders and upper back toward floor. To increase stretch of shoulders, keep forearms at same height on wall and move thighs backward.

☐ When shoulders feel stretched, push away from wall, lower arms to sides, and rest in upright position.

☐ This pose removes tightness and fatigue in upper back and shoulders.

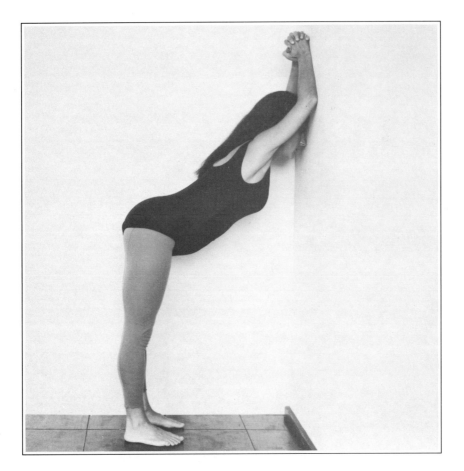

# Shoulder Stretch
# On Counter

☐ Place elbows securely on edge of counter or table. Position elbows no farther apart than width of shoulders.

☐ Walk feet back until legs are directly under hips and spine is parallel to floor. Press palms together and allow head to relax between arms.

☐ Inhale, tighten front thigh muscles, and lift buttock bones toward ceiling. Exhale and descend shoulders and spine toward floor. Continue to soften shoulder joints with each successive breath.

☐ To release, lower hands on counter, push back, stand upright, lower arms to sides, and rest.

☐ This posture stretches shoulders and lower back. It relieves abdominal pressure due to weight of uterus.

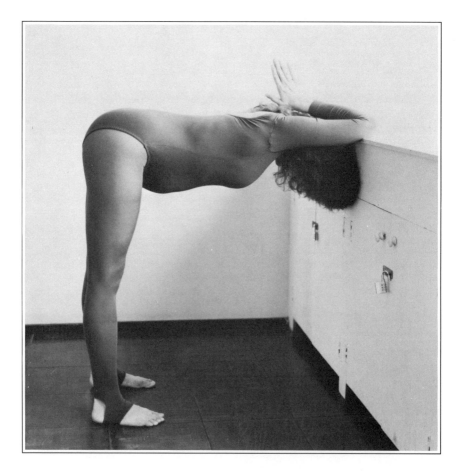

# Shoulder Stretch
# Kneeling To Wall

- [ ] Face wall, kneel 12 to 18 inches away from wall, bring feet together, and lower buttocks toward floor. Widen legs a comfortable distance apart and sit on heels.

- [ ] Stretch arms straight up wall. Place palms on wall, relax head between arms, and rest forehead on wall.

- [ ] To open shoulder area, reach up with straight arms while stretching upper body forward toward wall. Move tailbone downward to lessen curve in lower back. Let go of tightness in shoulders with each exhalation.

- [ ] To release, push away from wall, bring knees together, sit on heels, and relax arms to sides.

- [ ] This posture relieves shoulder stiffness, reduces upper back roundness, and opens rib cage.

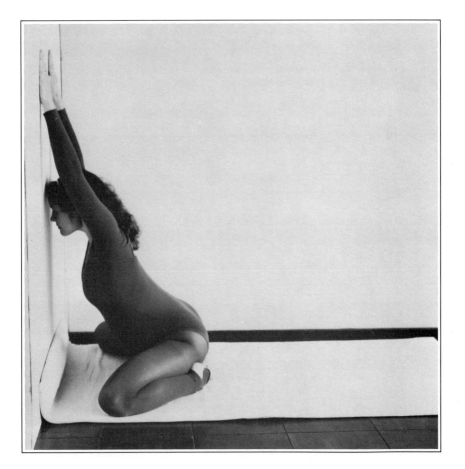

# Seated Shoulder Stretch

- ☐ Place front edge of chair seat 1 to 2 feet from wall. Sit on front half of chair with knees a comfortable distance apart. Turn feet out slightly.

- ☐ Extend arms straight up wall. Press buttocks firmly into chair, and allow forehead to rest on wall.

- ☐ Inhale and reach upward, exhale and stretch forward. To increase shoulder stretch, keep arms straight while stretching chest forward toward wall.

- ☐ Push away from wall, lean back in chair, relax arms at sides, and breathe normally.

- ☐ This pose stretches tight shoulders and opens chest. This passive posture is ideal during the third trimester of pregnancy.

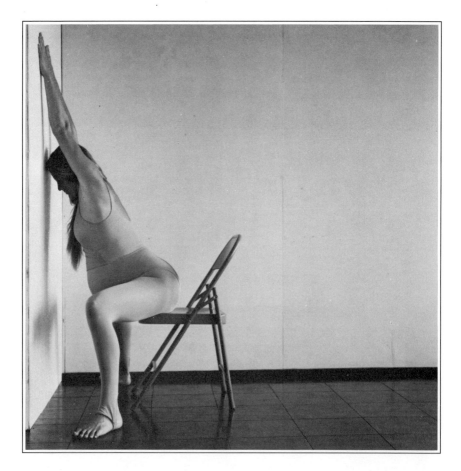

# Standing Shoulder Stretch To Wall

☐ Stretch arms straight up wall. Place palms flat on wall and walk feet back until legs are directly under hips. Position feet parallel to each other.

☐ To increase stretch in backs of legs, straighten legs and tighten front thigh muscles. Rest forehead on wall.

☐ Inhale and extend arms up wall. Exhale and stretch chest forward. To increase shoulder stretch, maintain height of palms on wall and move thighs backward. Breathe normally and relax shoulders and upper back.

☐ Release pose, stand upright, and relax arms to sides.

☐ This pose relieves stiffness in shoulders, upper back, and legs caused by sitting for a long time.

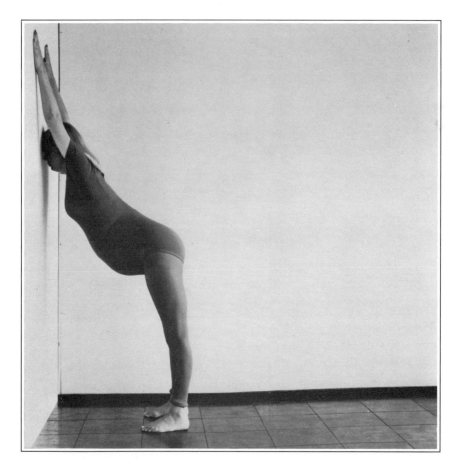

# Right Angle Pose
# To Wall

- [ ] Extend arms straight out from shoulders and place palms on wall. Walk feet back until arms and back are parallel to floor, and legs are directly under hips. Position feet parallel to each other, and stretch toes.

- [ ] To lengthen lower back, tighten front thigh muscles, push wall firmly, and extend hips away from wall. Keep head in line with arms, and fully stretch shoulders.

- [ ] Breathe naturally, lengthening torso with each exhalation. Hold pose until back feels stretched.

- [ ] Release arms, stand upright, and relax arms to sides.

- [ ] This posture relieves lower back tension. This pose is beneficial in the third trimester when heaviness of uterus causes lower back muscles to contract.

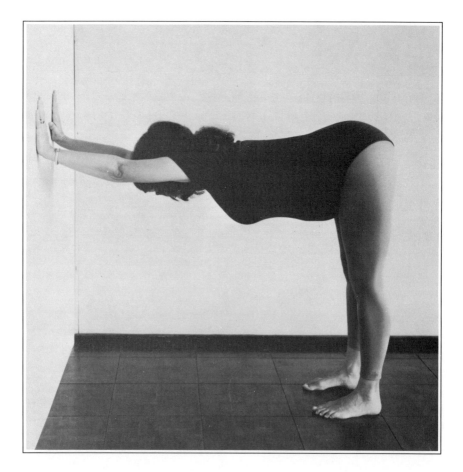

# Downward Dog
# Pose With Chair

- [ ] Push chair securely to wall. Grasp edges of chair seat firmly, or hook thumbs around front edge of seat and place palms on top of chair seat.

- [ ] Straighten arms and walk feet well back. Position parallel feet 8-12 inches apart. Tighten front thigh muscles, completely straighten legs, and lift buttock bones toward ceiling.

- [ ] Inhale and push down on chair seat to stretch arms and shoulders. Exhale and lengthen entire back away from hands. Breathe normally and descend head and chest.

- [ ] When back is extended, release, and stand upright.

- [ ] This pose relieves lower back tension, strengthens arms and back, and stretches hamstring and calf muscles.

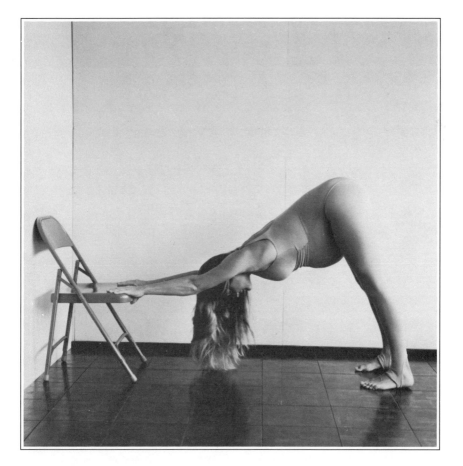

# Downward Dog Pose

- [ ] Kneel 3 to 3 1/2 feet in front of wall. Widen knees, sit back on heels, and extend arms toward wall. Place palms on floor and wedge thumbs and index fingers to wall.

- [ ] Come onto hands and knees. Keep weight on hands, turn toes under, and lift hips and knees off floor. Place parallel feet 8-12 inches apart, tighten front thigh muscles, straighten legs, and lift buttock bones.

- [ ] Inhale and stretch arms. Exhale, lengthen entire spine upwards, and press heels toward floor. A pillow may be placed under head for support and relaxation.

- [ ] To release, bend knees, sit back on heels, and rest.

- [ ] This posture strengthens arms and back, stretches hamstring and calf muscles, and relieves fatigue.

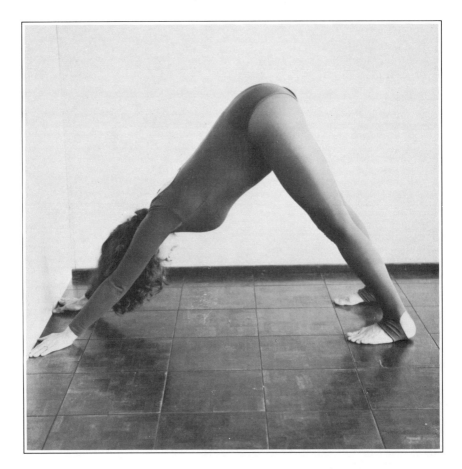

# Chest And Shoulder Stretch With Chair

- [ ] Place chair to wall and pad seat with pillow. Sit on blanket or pillow, extend arms behind back, rest arms on chair seat, and interlock fingers.

- [ ] If pose is difficult, raise buttocks with additional pillows, separate hands, and hold sides of chair seat. Widen feet slightly, straighten legs, and tighten front thigh muscles.

- [ ] Inhale, press backs of legs and buttocks to floor. Exhale, lift chest, and roll shoulders back. Breathe normally.

- [ ] To release, remove arms from chair seat, sit in a comfortable sitting position, and relax arms to sides.

- [ ] The posture stretches muscles of chest and shoulders, and helps relieve upper back roundness.

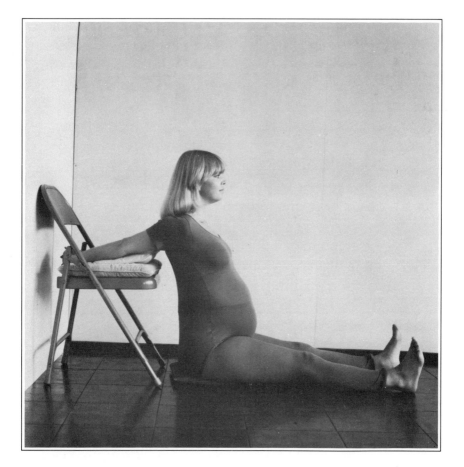

# Chapter 3

# THE STANDING POSES

The safest way to develop strength during pregnancy is to practice yoga's standing postures. Exercise during pregnancy must create strength as well as flexibility. The standing poses stretch *and* strengthen.

The standing poses are easily adapted for each trimester of pregnancy. They may be performed with the aid of a wall or chair during the third trimester.

Inactivity produces lethargy, standing poses develop vigor. They create energy because they increase circulation. These yoga poses expand the rib cage, deepen breathing, and develop stamina.

Muscle cramps are common in pregnancy. Regular practice of the standing poses may help relieve leg cramps by increasing circulation in the legs.

During pregnancy the additional weight of the uterus places added stress on the lower back. In any activity if the legs and hips are tight, the lower back must do more of the work. Stretching hip and leg muscles in the standing poses creates the mobility which lessens the stress on the lower back.

Standing postures create strong legs. As legs become stronger, leg fatigue lessens. Strong legs help position the pelvis and spinal column correctly. When the pelvis is positioned in a balanced way, there is less strain on the back. Strong legs and back are necessary to support the growing uterus.

It is the combination of strength and flexibility which takes the strain off the back in pregnancy. Practicing standing poses creates this healthful, pain-free balance.

# Hints And Cautions

Standing poses are strenuous and should not be held for a long time. During the first trimester, many pregnant women experience periods of fatigue and dizziness. Energetic standing poses would not be appropriate at these times.

In the third trimester, vigorous wide leg standing postures may place too much weight and pressure on the pelvic floor. The same postures may be performed safely using a chair for support.

During pregnancy a hormone called *relaxin* is secreted. This hormone has a loosening and softening effect on the ligaments. For this reason it is important not to overstretch when exercising. Overstretching ligaments may cause unstable joints. Relaxin may effect the sacroiliac joint and create discomfort in the standing postures.

One or both of the legs are kept straight throughout the following poses. It is important to learn how to correctly straighten the legs in order to create the maximum possible stability. Bend your knees slightly and place your fingers on your kneecaps. Tighten your front thigh muscles, the quadriceps, and feel the kneecaps lift. Maintain this lifted position whenever a pose calls for straight legs.

# Tree Pose

- [ ] Stand with back to wall and feet a few inches from wall. Transfer weight to right leg. Bend left knee and place left foot firmly on inside of right thigh or knee. Left toes point straight downward.

- [ ] Extend arms and place fingers on wall for support. Lift kneecap and thigh muscles of right leg. Balance weight evenly on right foot.

- [ ] Stretch chest, sides of body, and right thigh upward. If balance is secure, release fingers from wall and stretch arms above head. Look straight ahead.

- [ ] Release, lower leg and arms. Reverse pose bending right knee and balancing on left leg.

- [ ] Tree pose improves balance and strengthens legs.

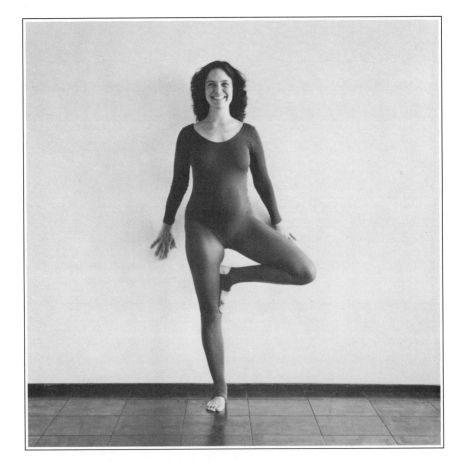

# Eagle Pose

☐ Stand with back to wall and feet a few inches from wall. Extend arms and place fingers to wall.

☐ Bend left leg with knee pointing straight ahead. Wrap right leg over left thigh and, if possible, hook toes behind left calf muscle.

☐ Lift the chest and balance body evenly over left leg. With fingers to wall for support, bend left knee and lower body slightly. Slowly straighten leg and release.

☐ To reverse pose, bend right leg, wrap left leg over right thigh and around right calf. Release pose, stand upright, and rest lower back to wall.

☐ This posture stretches hip muscles, strengthens thigh muscles, prevents calf cramps, and improves balance.

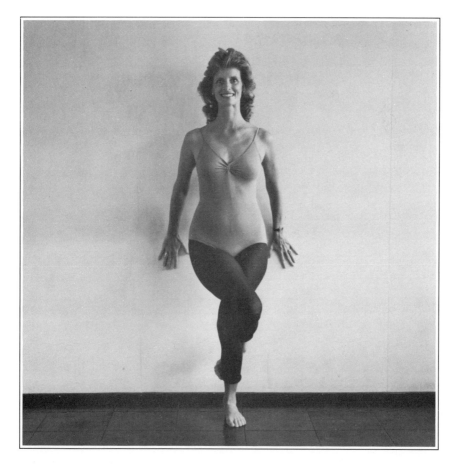

# Alternate Leg
# Stretch With Chair

- [ ] Place chair 4 to 5 feet away from wall. Stand with back to wall, position left heel to wall, and extend right foot 3 feet from wall. Left toes turn in slightly, and right toes point straight ahead.

- [ ] Place hands on hips and adjust left hip forward until both hips are parallel to chair. Inhale and lift chest. Exhale and bend forward at hips keeping back straight.

- [ ] Stretch arms forward and hold top of chair back. With each exhalation, stretch backs of legs by drawing up front thigh muscles and lifting buttock bones.

- [ ] When pose becomes easy, push chair foward, and stretch until chest is parallel to floor. Release and reverse with left foot forward.

- [ ] This pose stretches backs of legs, shoulders, and back.

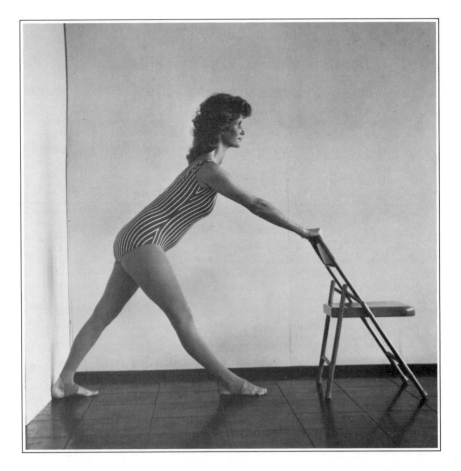

# Standing Alternate Leg Stretch

☐ Stand with back to wall. Place right heel to wall and take a 3-foot step forward with left foot. Align hips, lift thigh muscles, and point left toes straight forward.

☐ Press palms together behind back. Rotate hands until fingers point upward. Inhale and straighten legs. Exhale, bend forward at hips, and keep back straight.

☐ Tilt buttock bones upward and stretch breastbone forward until back is level with floor. Breathe normally and elongate spine with each exhalation.

☐ Release and reverse legs. After completing both sides, rest with back to wall and arms relaxed at sides.

☐ This pose loosens tight shoulders and wrists, stretches leg muscles, and improves posture.

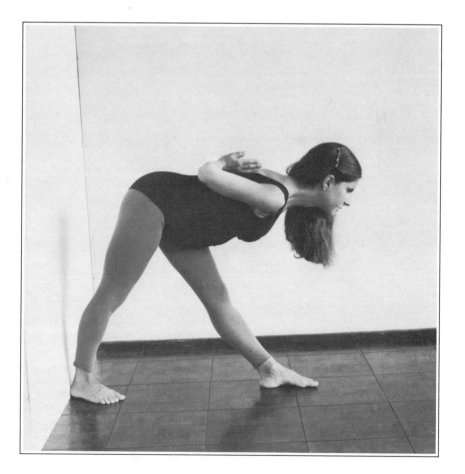

# Triangle Pose

☐ With right heel to wall, widen legs 3 to 4 feet apart. Turn left foot out 90 degrees. Align heel of left foot with arch of right foot. Rotate straight left leg outward to bring top thigh, knee, and foot in line.

☐ Press in with left hand at top of left thigh, tilt pelvis, and stretch upper body sideways to left. Keep both sides of torso evenly stretching. Lower left hand to left shin.

☐ Create firmness in legs and continue to extend left ribs laterally. On an exhalation stretch right arm vertically, rotate right hip and shoulder upward, and look toward right hand. Breathe normally.

☐ Release pose, change legs, and stretch to right.

☐ This pose strengthens legs, elongates spine, and stretches outer hip and inner thigh muscles.

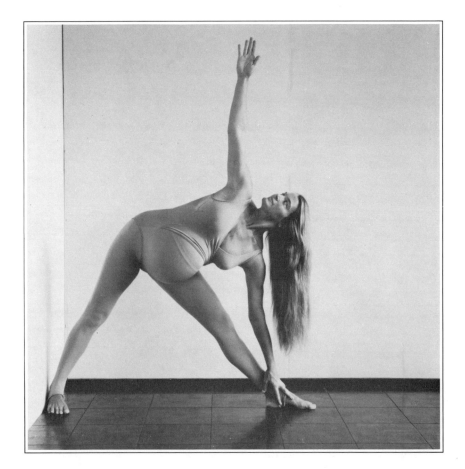

# Warrior II Pose
# To Wall

☐ Place right foot to wall and widen legs 4 to 4 1/2 feet apart. Turn left foot out 90 degrees, and align heel of left foot with arch of right foot.

☐ Keeping right leg straight, bend left knee until left thigh and shin bones create a right angle. Hold left knee back with left hand, and tuck tailbone under.

☐ To increase stretch across front pelvis, pull right hip back with right hand. Lift top chest, release hands from hips, and lift and extend arms straight out from shoulders. Hold this strenuous pose for a short time.

☐ Release pose, reverse legs, and bend right knee. After completing both sides, rest with back to wall.

☐ This pose opens groin area, strengthens legs, and creates endurance.

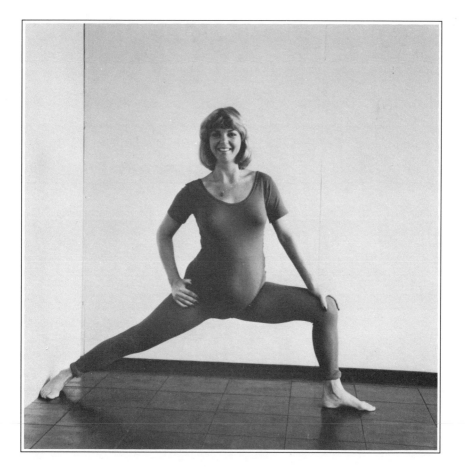

# Warrior II Pose
# With Chair

☐ Place chair to wall. Sit on chair with right buttock supported by chair seat. Bend right knee and align inner right thigh with front edge of chair seat.

☐ Extend left leg on floor and turn toes in slightly. Line up right heel with arch of left foot. Right toes point straight ahead and thigh and shin are perpendicular.

☐ While maintaining alignment of inner right thigh, stretch groin area by pulling back left hip. Lift both sides of chest evenly, relax shoulders, and tuck tailbone under. Breathe normally while stretching.

☐ Release and repeat pose to left. Complete both sides and rest sitting in chair with knees together.

☐ This pose stretches groin and inner thigh muscles.

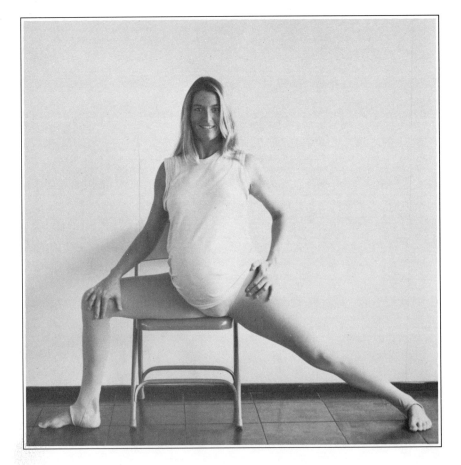

# Extended Warrior II
# Pose With Chair

☐ Place chair to wall. Sit on chair with left buttock supported by chair seat. Bend left knee and align inner left thigh with front edge of chair seat.

☐ Extend right leg on floor and turn toes in slightly. Line up left heel with arch of right foot. Left toes point straight ahead and thigh and shin are perpendicular.

☐ Raise arms and extend them straight out from shoulders. Lift breastbone and roll shoulders back and down. Turn head and look over left arm. Maintain even stretch of groin muscles and sides of body.

☐ Release, change legs, and do pose to right. Complete both sides, lower arms, and rest sitting in chair.

☐ This pose strengthens arms and improves posture.

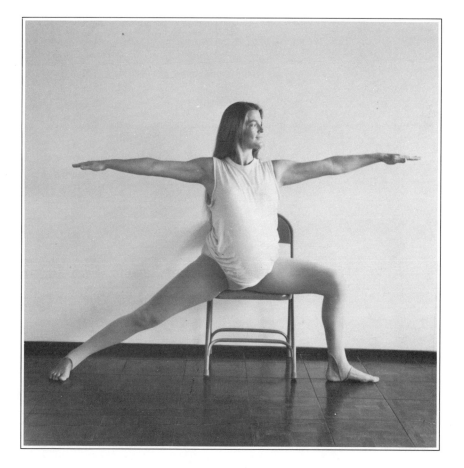

# Side Angle Pose
# To Wall

☐ Widen legs 4 to 4 1/2 feet apart and place right heel to wall. Turn left foot out 90 degrees, and align heel of left foot with arch of right foot.

☐ Keeping right leg straight, bend left knee until left thigh and shin form a right angle. Tilt pelvis to left and rest forearm on top of left thigh.

☐ Maintain alignment of left knee and pull right hip back to increase stretch across front pelvis. With each exhalation roll right shoulder back, tuck left buttock under, and extend sides of body evenly to left.

☐ Release pose, change legs, and extend body to right. After completing both sides, rest in upright position.

☐ This posture lengthens sides of body and stretches inner thigh, groin, and back muscles.

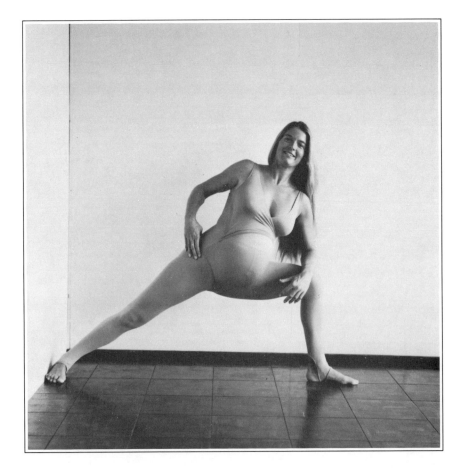

# Side Angle Pose
# With Chair

- [ ] Place chair to wall. Sit on chair with right buttock supported by chair seat. Bend right knee and align inner right thigh with front edge of chair seat.

- [ ] Extend left leg on floor and grip floor with slightly turned in toes. Align right heel with arch of left foot. Right thigh and shin form a right angle.

- [ ] Extend both sides of body to right. Hold right knee in position and pull back left hip to increase stretch between hips. Stretch left arm diagonally overhead with palm facing down. Turn head and look over left shoulder.

- [ ] Release and repeat pose to left. Complete both sides and rest sitting in chair with knees together.

- [ ] This posture stretches arms, inner thighs, and spine.

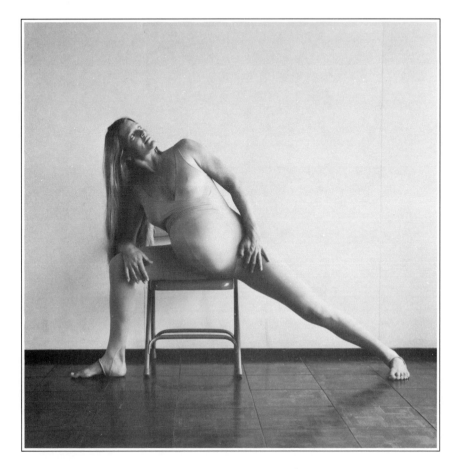

# Half Moon Pose
# With Wall

☐ Stand with back to wall, place right heel to side wall, and widen feet 3 to 3 1/2 feet apart or length of one leg. Point left toes ahead with foot 2 inches from wall.

☐ Place books or bench to wall 9-12 inches ahead of left foot. Bend left knee, shift weight to left foot, rest hand on books, lift right leg up wall, and place sole of foot on side wall. Adjust balancing leg until directly under hip.

☐ Fully stretch both legs. Lean buttocks on wall and roll right hip up to stretch across front pelvis. Adjust books until left arm is under shoulder and then raise right arm straight up. Breathe and extend spine.

☐ To release, bend left knee, set right foot on floor, and stand upright. Reverse pose bending to right.

☐ This pose improves balance and opens hip area.

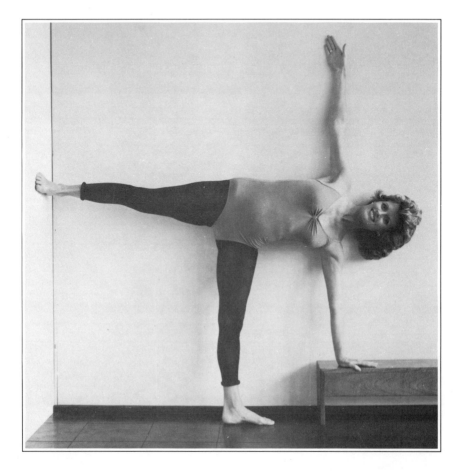

# Warrior I Pose
# To Wall

☐ Place right toes to wall. Stretch left leg back 4 feet. Lift left heel, come onto ball of foot, and move left hip slightly forward until both hips are parallel to wall.

☐ Place fingertips on wall in line with shoulders. Inhale and lift chest. Exhale and bend right knee until thigh and shin form a right angle.

☐ Tuck tailbone firmly to lessen lower back arch. Push away from wall and stretch breastbone toward ceiling. If balance is secure, raise both arms overhead.

☐ To release, lower arms, and straighten right leg. Repeat pose with left leg to wall and right leg extended. After completing both sides, rest in upright position.

☐ This posture stretches and strengthens thigh muscles and creates stamina.

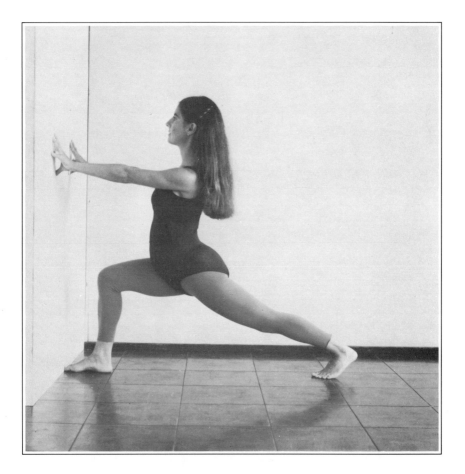

# Wide Leg Stretch
# To Wall

☐ Stand with back to wall. Separate legs 4 feet apart. Place feet parallel and 2 inches from wall. Keep back straight, bend forward from hips, and place fingertips on floor under shoulders. If back rounds trying to reach floor, elevate hands on books or chair.

☐ Inhale, fully straighten legs, lift back thighs up wall, and spread buttock bones apart. Exhale, press buttocks to wall, release spine straight out of pelvis, and stretch chest forward. Breathe and extend spine.

☐ To release, bend knees slightly, lean back on wall, and come to upright position. Bring legs together and rest with lower back pressed to wall. Breathe normally.

☐ This pose lessons fatigue and stretches inner thigh, back, and hamstring muscles.

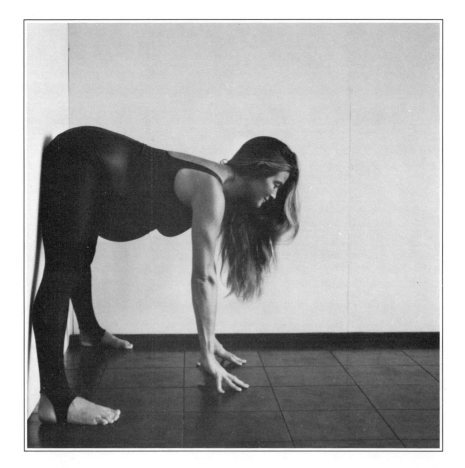

# Head To Floor
# Wide Leg Stretch

☐ Stand with back to wall and separate feet 4 feet apart. Align feet parallel to each other. Bend forward from hips and place hands on floor in line with feet.

☐ Tighten front thigh muscles, turn toes slightly inward, and grip floor firmly with feet. Allow back leg muscles to stretch and release spine downward.

☐ If backs of legs stretch easily, allow head to touch floor. Interlock fingers behind head and place hands and forearms on floor.

☐ Inhale and press downward with feet and forearms. Exhale and stretch back thighs, buttocks, and spine upward. Release pose and rest in upright position.

☐ This pose stretches hamstring and inner thigh muscles.

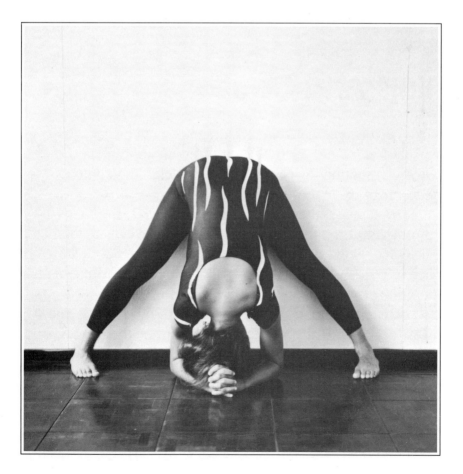

# Chapter 4

# THE FRONT HIP AND THIGH STRETCHING POSES

Activities such as jogging, bicycling, walking, sitting, and climbing stairs tighten the front hip and thigh muscles. Very few everyday activities stretch these muscles. Tight muscles on the front of the hip, combined with the added weight of the uterus, pull the front pelvis downward. This may cause pain and compression in the lower back.

Front hip and thigh stretches counterbalance the squatting and hip stretching poses in Chapter 5 and the hamstring stretching poses in Chapter 6. Together these poses create an even development of legs and hips, and a feeling of freedom in the joints.

The hero's pose and variations have a revitalizing effect on legs, feet, and ankles. Sitting in the hero's pose improves circulation in legs, removes fatigue, and lessens swelling in ankles.

# Hints And Cautions

When performing the front thigh lunges on one knee, keep the pelvis level and the tailbone tucked under to prevent overstretching the lower abdominal muscles and compressing the lower back.

These poses intensely stretch the knees. If the knees are stiff or painful in the hero's pose, sufficiently elevate the buttocks with folded blankets. If the tops of the feet are painful, place rolled towels under the ankles for comfort. Move in and out of the poses slowly to prevent straining the knees.

After performing the reclining hero's pose, widen the knees, bend forward, and rest the forehead on the mat. This position lengthens lower back muscles. Then sit and completely extend the legs.

# Hero's Pose

☐ Kneel on mat or blanket. Separate feet, place hands on floor for support, lower buttocks carefully between heels, and sit on pillow or folded blanket.

☐ Adjust height under buttocks for comfort. Stretch feet straight back and pad ankles if tops of feet are not comfortable. Stretch should be felt in thighs, not knees.

☐ Squeeze knees toward each other, press down on floor with fingertips, and stretch spine upward. Rest palms on knees and lift and expand chest with each breath.

☐ Widen knees, sit on heels, bend forward, and rest head on floor with arms to sides. Release and extend legs.

☐ Hero's pose relieves leg fatigue, stretches front thighs and insteps, and may prevent varicose veins.

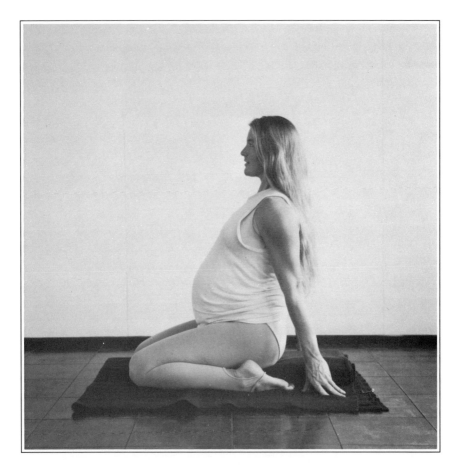

# Hero's Pose With Arms Overhead

☐ Kneel on mat. Widen feet, support body weight with hands, and lower buttocks onto folded blanket or pillow.

☐ Stretch feet straight back and bring knees closer together. Adjust height under buttocks if necessary. If buttocks touch floor easily, remove pillow.

☐ Inhale, interlock fingers, and lift chest. Exhale and stretch arms overhead with palms facing toward ceiling. Extend arms upward from shoulder blades. Maintain straightness of spine and lift upward from lower back.

☐ Lower arms to sides. Widen knees, bend forward, place folded forearms on floor and rest with head on forearms. After releasing pose, straighten and extend both legs.

☐ This pose stretches thighs and helps relieve indigestion.

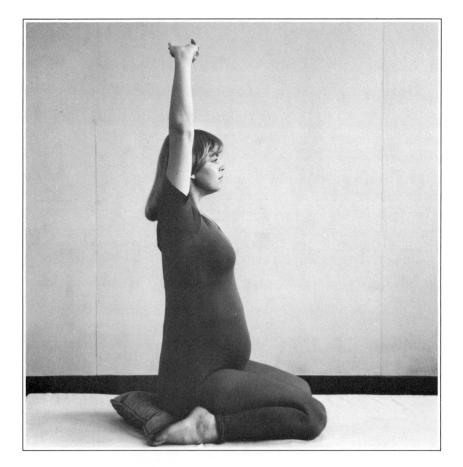

# Half Reclining
# Hero's Pose

☐ Place stack of blankets or firm pillows behind back. Kneel on mat. Separate feet, support weight of body with hands, and lower buttocks carefully between heels onto pillow. Adjust height under buttocks for comfort.

☐ Squeeze knees closer together and stretch feet straight back alongside hips. Lean back and rest lower forearms on pillows. Look straight ahead.

☐ To lengthen lower back, press down firmly on pillows, elongate spine, and lift chest. Concentrate on expanding rib cage with each breath.

☐ To release, sit upright, bend forward, lower forehead onto folded arms, and rest. Sit up and extend legs.

☐ This posture helps improve breathing, and stretches muscles of insteps, front thighs, and chest.

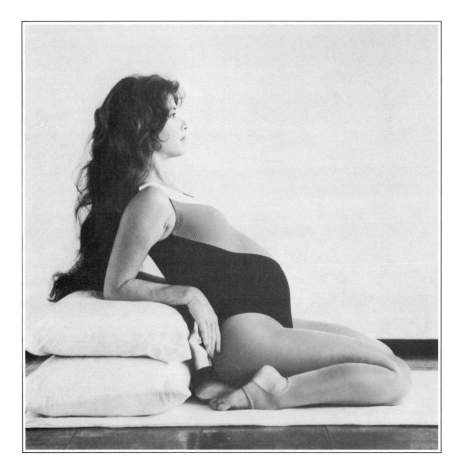

# Reclining Hero Pose

☐ For a first trimester student with front thigh flexibility.

☐ Arrange pillows to form a wedge shape. Kneel with back to pillows, separate feet, support body weight with hands, and lower buttocks onto mat.

☐ Stretch feet straight back alongside hips and squeeze knees closer together. Place narrow edge of pillow wedge to tailbone. Lower spine onto pillows, support head with small pillow, and relax arms on mat.

☐ Close eyes and deepen breath. Concentrate on expanding chest with each breath. To release, press down with hands, lift chest, and sit upright. Bend forward and rest forehead on folded arms. Sit up and extend legs.

☐ This pose stretches front thighs and improves digestion.

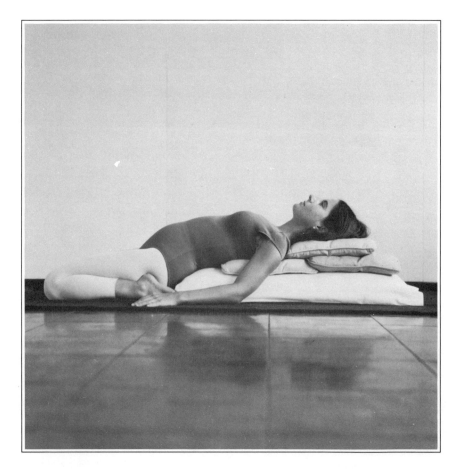

# Reclining Alternate Front Thigh Stretch

- [ ] For a first trimester student with front thigh flexibility.

- [ ] Arrange pillows to form a wedge shape. Sit with back to pillows and legs extended. Fold left lower leg straight back with foot alongside hip. Align pillows to tailbone.

- [ ] Recline and rest spine on pillows, support head with small pillow, and relax arms on mat. Extend and straighten right leg. Right toes and knee face ceiling. Or right knee may be bent and sole of right foot placed on mat.

- [ ] Relax left thigh and spine. Expand rib cage sideways with each breath. To come up, press down with forearms, lift chest, and sit upright. Reverse pose, bend right leg back, straighten left, and recline. Release and extend both legs.

- [ ] This pose alternately stretches front thigh muscles.

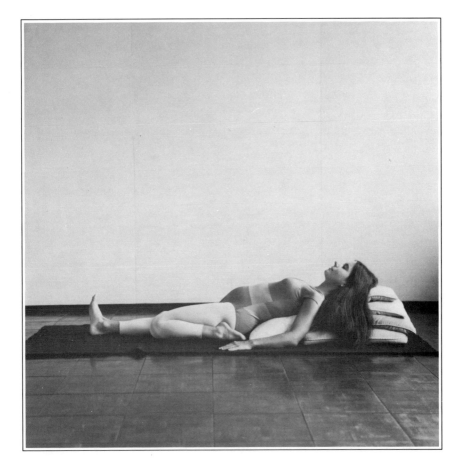

# Standing Front Thigh Stretch With Chair

- [ ] Stand behind chair. Hold top of chair back for support with left hand. Shift weight onto straight left leg. Bend right knee and lift foot toward buttock. Hold instep of right foot with right hand.

- [ ] Inhale and lift chest. Exhale, tuck tailbone under, and tighten left thigh muscles. Bend elbow and pull right foot closer to right buttock to stretch thigh muscles. Right kneecap faces floor.

- [ ] Release right foot and lower leg. Reverse pose, hold chair with right hand, bend left knee, and hold left foot. After completing both sides, stand upright, hold onto chair back, and breathe normally.

- [ ] This pose aids balance, strengthens straight leg, and stretches front thigh muscles of bent leg.

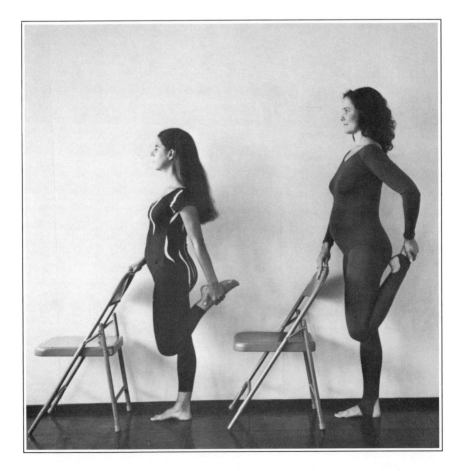

# Kneeling Front Thigh Stretch With Chair

- [ ] Place chair to wall. Kneel on mat with left knee on pillow. Lift right knee and place right foot on mat with toes under chair. Right shin and thigh form right angle.

- [ ] Align right knee or shin with front edge of chair seat. Press down on chair seat, lift chest, and elongate spine.

- [ ] Lift front hipbones vertically and move tailbone downward towards floor. While maintaining lift of chest and tuck of tailbone, slide left knee slightly backward. Stretch will be felt in center of thigh muscles.

- [ ] Change legs, placing right knee on pillow, and left knee to edge of chair seat. Release and sit on mat in comfortable cross-legged pose.

- [ ] This pelvic tilting pose stretches groin and thigh muscles.

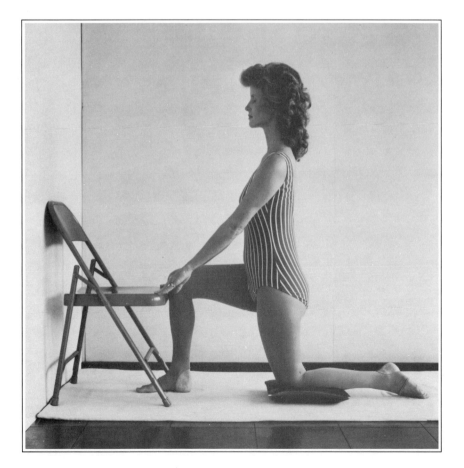

# Kneeling Front Thigh Stretch

☐ Kneel on mat with right knee on pillow. Lift left knee, extend lower leg forward, and place sole of left foot on mat. Left thigh and shin form a right angle.

☐ Place hands on hips and lengthen lower back by tucking tailbone under and lifting front hipbones. Inhale and lift top chest and elongate spine. Exhale and gradually bend left knee straight forward.

☐ Keep tailbone tucked to restrict stretch to front thigh and groin muscles. Gently increase stretch with each breath. Interlock fingers behind back and extend arms.

☐ Reverse pose, placing left knee on pillow, and right foot on floor. Release and rest in comfortable sitting position.

☐ This pose stretches groin and thigh muscles.

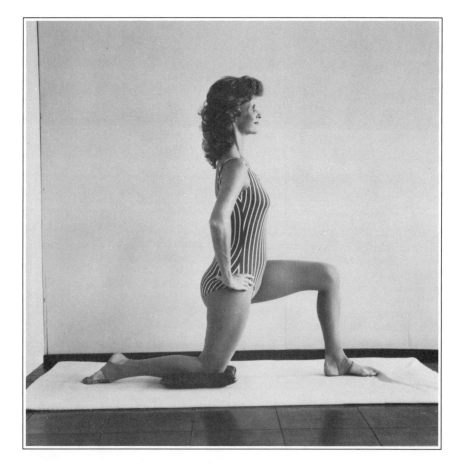

# Intense Front Thigh Stretch To Wall

☐ For a first trimester student with front thigh flexibility.

☐ Place right knee on pillow to wall. Stretch lower leg straight up wall with toes pointing toward ceiling.

☐ Bring left leg forward until left thigh and shin form a right angle and toes point straight forward. Extend arms and place palms on wall. Breathe and stretch upward.

☐ Lengthen lower back by tucking tailbone under and lifting front hipbones. Inhale, lift chest, and elongate spine. Exhale and move right hip away from wall to increase stretch in front thigh muscles.

☐ Reverse pose, placing left knee on pillow and right foot on floor. Release and rest in comfortable sitting position.

☐ This pose stretches front thigh muscles intensely.

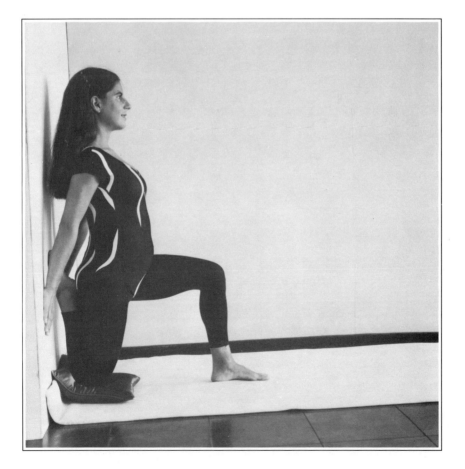

# Seated Alternate Front Thigh Stretch

- [ ] Sit on mat with legs outstretched. Bend right knee and fold right lower leg straight back with foot alongside hip.

- [ ] Elevate left buttock with pillow and straighten left leg. To increase stretch in hamstrings, tighten left front thigh muscles, extend left heel, and stretch toes toward ceiling.

- [ ] Place hands on floor alongside hips and lift chest. Bend forward slightly from hips keeping back straight. Concentrate on upward lift of spine and maintenance of normal spinal curves.

- [ ] Reverse pose, bend left lower leg back, and straighten right leg. Release and extend both legs.

- [ ] This pose stretches hamstring muscles of one leg while stretching front thigh muscles of other leg.

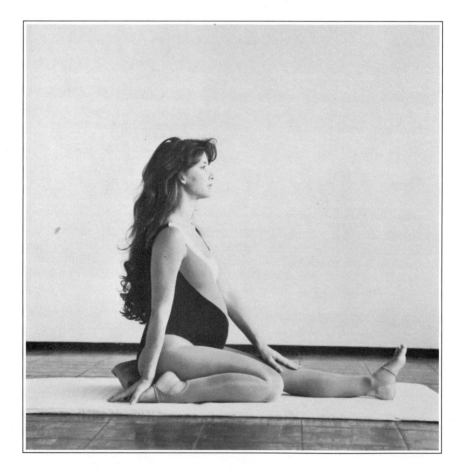

# Alternate Front Thigh Stretch With Chair

- ☐ Sit in front of chair placed on mat. Bend right knee and fold right lower leg straight back with foot alongside hip.

- ☐ Elevate left buttock with pillow and extend left leg under chair. Pull chair closer until foot touches lower rung. Tighten left front thigh muscles to stretch hamstrings.

- ☐ Hold chair seat or sides of chair back firmly. Bend forward from hips and elongate spine. Raise hands higher up chair back and stretch chest forward. Intensify stretch of left leg by extending heel under chair rung.

- ☐ Reverse pose, bend left lower leg beside hip, and straighten right leg. Release and extend both legs.

- ☐ This pose elongates spine and alternately stretches front thigh and hamstring muscles.

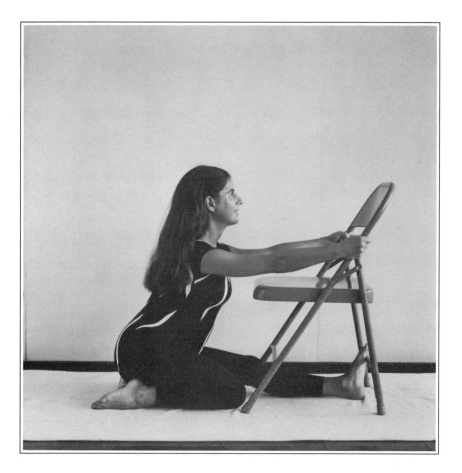

# Elevated Leg And Front Thigh Stretch

- [ ] Sit on small pillow 2 to 3 feet from wall. Bend left knee and fold left lower leg back with foot alongside hip.

- [ ] Lean back onto palms. Lift right leg and place right foot onto wall. Inhale, elongate spine, and lift chest. Exhale and tighten front thigh muscles of right leg on wall.

- [ ] Adjust distance from wall to increase or decrease stretch in legs. Maintain normal spinal curves by adjusting torso forward or backward. Extend heel on wall and flex toes.

- [ ] Lower leg from wall and reverse pose. Bend right lower leg beside hip, and place left foot on wall. Release pose.

- [ ] Elevating legs on wall reduces fatigue and may prevent swelling and leg cramps. Front thigh stretching also prevents thigh cramps by increasing circulation.

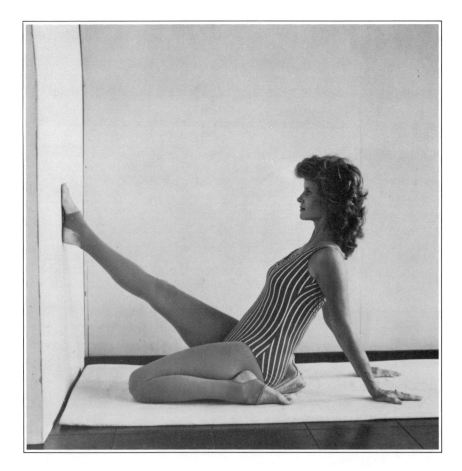

# Chapter 5

# THE SQUATTING AND HIP STRETCHING POSES

Stretching the muscles around the hip joint is an excellent preparation for labor. The bound angle pose and squatting pose can be used as actual labor positions.

These poses are effective when they are performed with breathing awareness. Remember to move on an exhalation. Hold the new position for a few breaths before increasing the stretch. Be patient and allow the muscles to release slowly.

The introduction to Chapter 1 stated that the position of the pelvis determines the curves of the spine. The balance of the muscles, tendons, and ligaments determines the tilt of the pelvis. The varied postures in this section develop the flexibility needed to keep the pelvis upright and the lower back pain free.

Performing the squatting poses (pp. 56-58) regularly opens the *pubic symphysis*, the junction of the pubic bones, which may facilitate labor.

*Sciatica*, an inflammation of the sciatic nerve causing pain down the back of the thigh, is common during pregnancy. The roots of the sciatic nerve originate in the lumbar and sacral vertebrae and pass down the back of the thigh. Sciatica during pregnancy has many causes. Supporting the added weight of the uterus may create tightness in the lower back, side of the hips, and buttocks. If sciatica is caused by tightness in these muscles, then the leg over leg stretch (p. 63) may alleviate the pain.

# Hints And Cautions

To avoid overstretching the ligaments, stretch the muscles of the hips slowly and carefully.

Do not remain in the squatting pose for a long time. Move in and out of the pose during labor. The downward pressure may cause nerve compression. Stretch out the legs between contractions.

# Half Squatting
# Pose To Wall

☐ Stand with back to wall. Place buttocks to wall, bend knees, separate feet, and move feet forward.

☐ Increase bend in knees, squat down until thighs are almost parallel to floor, feet are flat on floor, and legs are a comfortable distance from wall.

☐ Place elbows and forearms on inner thighs. Inhale and gently press knees apart. Exhale and lengthen spine forward away from wall. Hold until back feels stretched.

☐ Release, stand upright, and rest with back pressed to wall. In last trimester, perform pose while sitting on front edge of chair seat, widen thighs with forearms, and lift and lengthen spine away from chair seat.

☐ This posture strengthens front thigh muscles, stretches inner thigh muscles, and elongates spine.

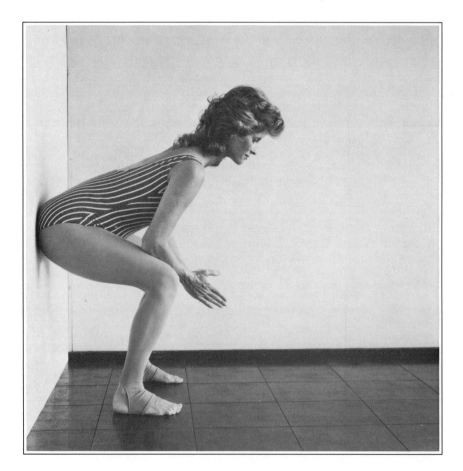

# Supported Squatting Pose

☐ Sit on firm pillow or stack of blankets. Widen knees apart and turn feet out.

☐ Place elbows to inner thighs and press palms together. Inhale and press elbows sideways. Exhale and relax inner thigh muscles. Lift chest and elongate spine.

☐ When stretch becomes easy, widen legs and increase outward pressure of elbows on inner thighs.

☐ Hold squat for 2 minutes. Release pose and fully extend both legs. Lean back on hands and relax top groin area.

☐ After standing or walking, supported squatting brings relaxation. During pregnancy squatting helps pelvic floor muscles to relax. Squatting during labor, with support of pillows or labor coach, may facilitate birth.

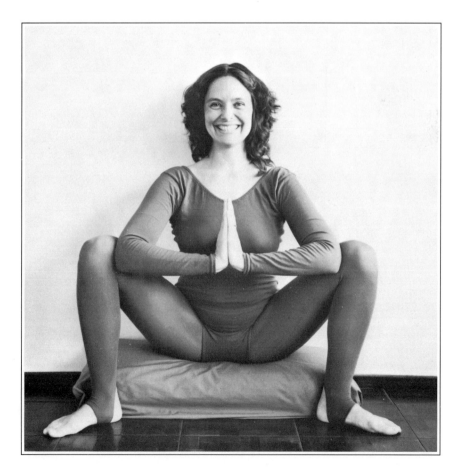

# Squatting Pose
# To Wall

☐ Stand with back to wall. Separate feet, bend knees, and squat with back resting on wall.

☐ Widen knees and turn feet outward for stability. Place elbows to inner knees and press palms together.

☐ Inhale and press knees apart with elbows. Exhale and stretch spine up wall. Allow tailbone to move toward floor and muscles of lower back to relax.

☐ Hold pose for 2-3 minutes. Release, sit on floor, stretch out both legs, and allow inner thighs to relax.

☐ Squatting stretches calf muscles and inner thigh muscles. Lower back muscles are stretched and backache is relieved. Squatting may facilitate labor by helping to open the pubic symphysis in the pelvis.

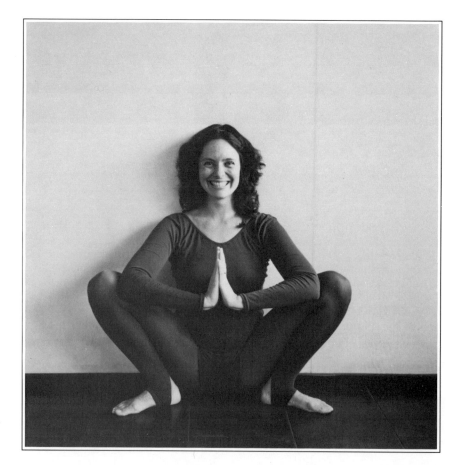

# Bound Angle Pose

☐ Pose may be done on rug or with back to wall. Sit on small pillow or folded blanket. Bend knees outward and press soles of feet together. Hold ankles and draw feet in as close as possible to pelvic floor.

☐ Place hands on floor beside hips. Inhale and lift entire spine upward. Exhale, relax inner thigh muscles, and release knees downward toward floor.

☐ Place palms on inner thighs. With an exhalation, press thighs gently toward floor to increase inner thigh stretch.

☐ When stretch becomes easy, bend forward from hips, maintain straightness of spine, and extend hands forward on floor. To release, sit upright and extend both legs.

☐ This pose increases hip flexibility, stretches inner thigh muscles, and is a comfortable position during labor.

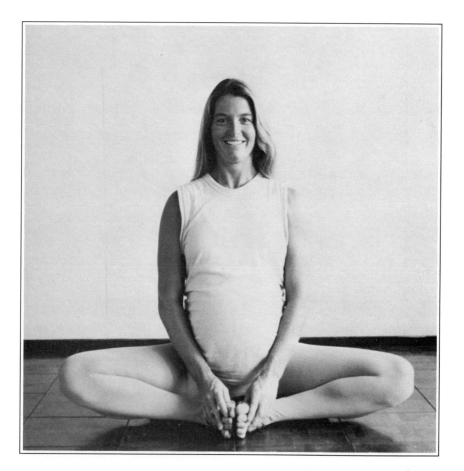

# Hip Stretch With Feet On Wall

☐ Place wedge shaped stack of pillows 1 1/2 to 2 feet from wall. Lie on pillows with narrow edge of wedge against tailbone. Pillows lift head and torso higher than hips.

☐ Bend and widen knees. Turn feet out slightly and place feet flat on wall. Adjust distance from wall and space between feet for comfort and stretch.

☐ To increase stretch in hip joints, lower feet toward floor. Place hands on inner knees and gently press knees toward floor. Perform each stretching movement on an exhalation. Concentrate on relaxing hip joints.

☐ To release, bend knees to chest, roll over onto one side, sit up, and rest in a comfortable sitting position.

☐ This pose prepares for labor by stretching hip muscles.

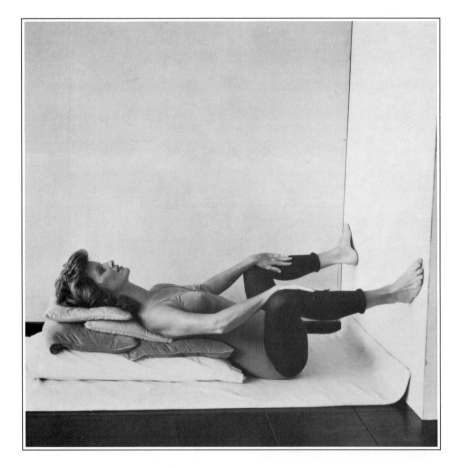

# Reclining Knee To Floor Pose

☐ Lie on wedge-shaped pillow pile with narrow edge of wedge against tailbone. Support head with small pillow.

☐ Bend left knee and hold left foot with both hands. Straighten and extend right leg on mat. Right thigh rolls inward, and right knee and toes face ceiling.

☐ Inhale and lift left foot until bottom of foot faces ceiling. On an exhalation descend left knee toward floor beside body. While stretching, maintain alignment of right leg.

☐ Release and extend left leg. Bend right knee and pull foot toward floor. After completing both sides, bend knees, roll onto one side, and come up to a sitting position.

☐ This pose increases rotation of thigh bones in hip sockets and stretches back thigh muscles.

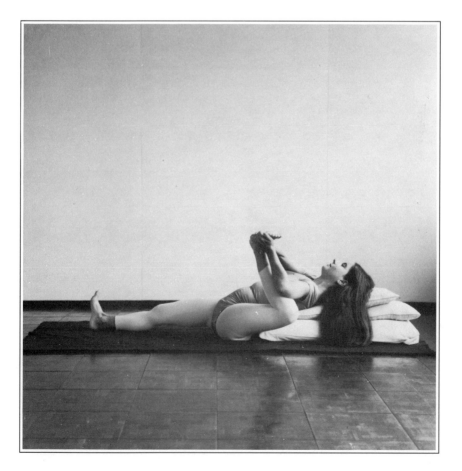

# Reclining Shin To Chest Pose

☐ Lie on wedge-shaped pillow pile with narrow end of wedge against tailbone. Support head with small pillow.

☐ Bend right knee and hold outer side of right shin with both hands. Hold above ankle bone and relax right foot. Straighten left leg on mat. Extend left foot and adjust leg until toes and knee face ceiling.

☐ Inhale and lift right foot until right shin is parallel to floor. Exhale and pull shin closer toward chest. Stretch will be felt in right hip and back thigh muscles.

☐ Release and extend right leg. Bend left knee and pull shin toward chest. After completing both sides, bend knees, roll onto one side, and sit upright in a comfortable pose.

☐ This posture stretches back thigh muscles and increases hip joint flexibility.

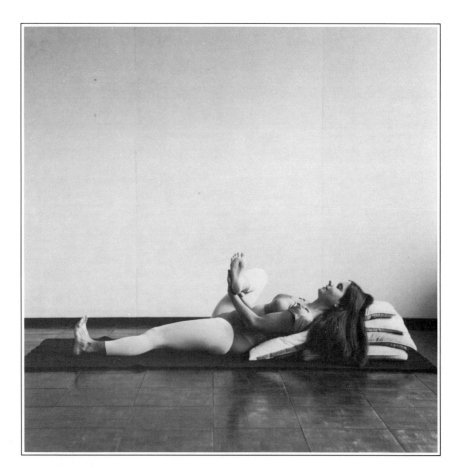

# Leg Over Leg Hip Stretch

☐ Sit on mat with legs outstretched. Bend both legs, place feet on floor. Fold left leg under right. Cross right leg over left. Align knees one over the other in line with navel. If hips are tight, knees may not touch each other. Elevate buttocks on pillow if necessary.

☐ Lean back on hands, press down, and lift chest and spine. To increase hip stretch, lean back on left hand and gently press right knee toward floor.

☐ When pose becomes easy, cross forearms and press down on right leg. To add a twisting movement, place left hand to outer right thigh, right hand on floor, lift chest, and twist torso toward right. Release and reverse position of legs.

☐ After completing both sides, extend legs and rest.

☐ This pose stretches sides of hips and may relieve sciatica.

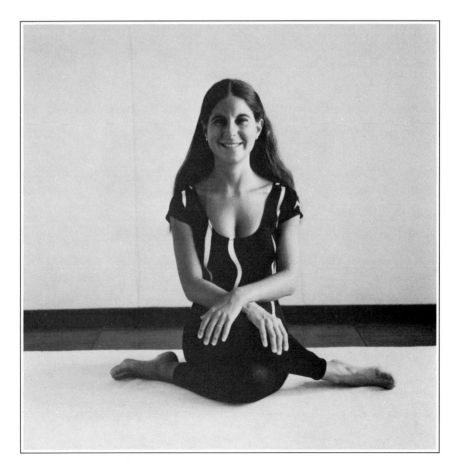

# Shoulder Stretches In Leg Over Leg Pose

☐ Sit on mat and cross right leg over left. To perform shoulder stretch shown on left, raise right arm, bend elbow, and place right hand in center of upper back.

☐ Bend left elbow, slide back of left hand up back and attempt to clasp hands. Hold belt between hands if necessary. Release and reverse arms. Release legs and relax both arms at sides.

☐ To perform shoulder stretch shown on right, sit on mat and cross left leg over right. Interlock fingers and stretch arms straight overhead. Turn palms toward ceiling, lift arms out of shoulder joints, and stretch back muscles.

☐ Lower arms, reverse interlock of fingers, and stretch arms straight overhead. Release legs and relax arms.

☐ These stretches remove shoulder joint stiffness.

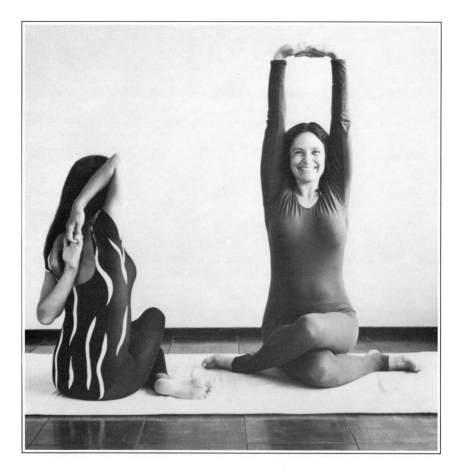

# Intense Hip Stretch

☐ Hip flexibility is necessary for comfort in this posture. Sit on mat with legs extended. Bend left knee and form a right angle with left thigh and shin.

☐ Bend right knee, and place right shin directly on top of left shin. Extend right foot beyond left knee and flex both feet. If pose is difficult, move left foot closer to body.

☐ Gently press right knee toward floor. Stretch will be felt deep within hip socket. Inhale and lift chest. Exhale and relax hip joints.

☐ Release pose and extend legs. Cross left shin over right. After stretching both sides, extend legs and rest.

☐ This posture stretches outer buttock muscles and increases hip joint flexibility.

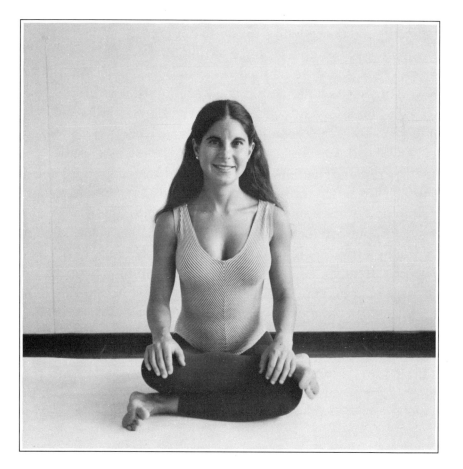

# Chapter 6

# THE HAMSTRING, CALF, & INNER THIGH STRETCHING POSES

Tight hamstring muscles aren't particularly noticeable until a pregnant women bends forward at the hips. Because tight back thigh muscles make bending forward difficult and even painful, most of the bend is taken instead by the flexible lower back. For the pregnant woman this means added strain on the back muscles. The lower back muscles are already overworked by having to support the growing uterus. Therefore, gradually stretching the hamstring muscles will relieve stress on the vulnerable lower back, and make freedom of forward movement possible.

The hamstring muscles on the back of the thigh are strong, stretch resistant muscles. They need to be worked patiently and consistently for maximum results. The hamstring muscles originate on the sitting bones (ischia) and insert below the knee on the lower leg bones (tibia and fibula). They cross both the hip and knee joints. Therefore, they are most intensely stretched when bending forward at the hips with completely straight legs.

The calf muscles are shortened by physical activities such as running, dancing, bicycling, and wearing high-heeled shoes. These tight muscles are particularly susceptible to cramping during pregnancy. Muscle cramping has many causes. Some are thought to be dietary. Another cause is poor circulation or pooling of blood in the legs. Cramps frequently occur at night, and calf stretches will help relieve them. At the first sign of a cramp, immediately flex the foot, draw the toes back toward the knee, and extend the heel.

Stretched inner thigh muscles may aid relaxation during labor. Learning to release the inner thighs has the physiological effect of softening the muscles and the psychological effect of relinquishing fear.

# Hints And Cautions

Develop the habit of using hamstring stretches as an antidote to lengthy periods of sitting. Stand up, face the chair, alternately place the heel of one foot on the chair seat, and gradually bend forward from the hips keeping the legs and back straight. This will negate the effects of sitting by increasing circulation and stretching the entire back leg.

Stretch hamstring and inner thigh muscles slowly and consistently. They will tear if stretched aggressively and are very slow to heal. Begin with the back-lying stretches in the first trimester. When performing seated poses, elevate the buttocks sufficiently to allow the forward movement to originate from the hips instead of the lower back. Use the leverage and support of a chair on the mat.

In addition, the standing poses in Chapter 2 are excellent poses for increasing hamstring, calf, and inner thigh flexibility.

# Reclining Alternate Leg Hamstring Stretch

☐ Arrange pillows to form a wedge shape. Sit in front of pillows with narrow edge of wedge against tailbone.

☐ Lie back onto pillows and support head with small pillow. Extend both legs on mat. Bend left knee, place belt around ball of foot, and straighten left leg.

☐ Extend and straighten right leg on mat. Right toes and knee face ceiling. Inhale and hold belt on left foot with both hands. Exhale and gently draw left leg toward chest. Maintain straightness of both legs during stretch.

☐ Bend left knee and release. Change legs and draw right leg toward chest. Release legs, roll onto one side, and sit up.

☐ This pose stretches hamstring and calf muscles. When hamstrings are stretched, back tension is lessened.

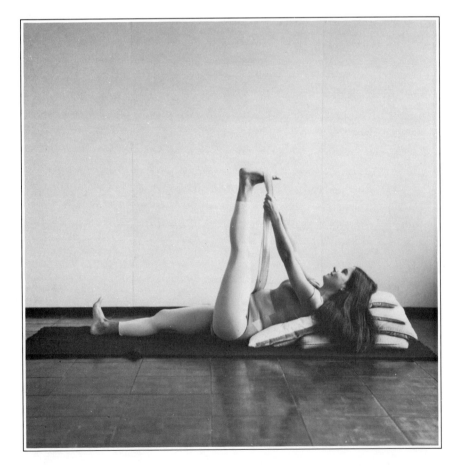

# Reclining Alternate Leg To Side Stretch

☐ Arrange pillows to form a wedge shape. Sit in front of pillows with legs extended. Recline and rest spine on pillows and support head with small pillow.

☐ Bend left knee and place strap around bottom of foot. Extend and straighten right leg on mat. Right toes and knee face ceiling. Extend right arm sideways on floor.

☐ Hold strap with left hand and straighten left leg. With leg straight, gradually open left leg sideways. Press downward on right hip to keep pelvis level.

☐ To release, bend left knee and lower leg. Reverse legs and open right leg sideways. After stretching both legs sideways, bend knees, roll onto one side, and sit up.

☐ This pose stretches hamstring and inner thigh muscles.

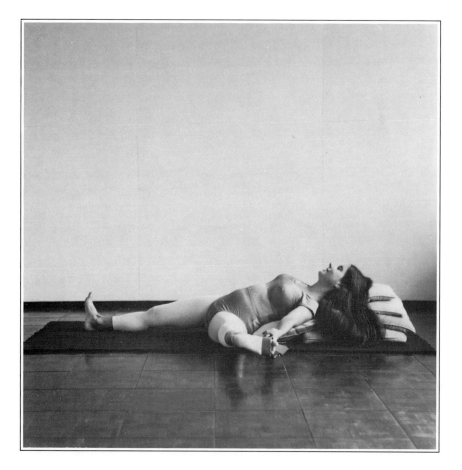

# Easy Hamstring Stretch In Chair

☐ Place chair to wall and small pillow on floor. Sit on front edge of chair seat and hold sides of chair seat.

☐ Bend left knee and place foot flat on floor. Extend right leg and rest heel on pillow on floor. Press down on chair seat, or stretch arms backward and hold sides of chair.

☐ Inhale, bend forward slightly from hips, lift chest, and elongate spine. Exhale, extend right heel, and pull toes backward toward knee.

☐ To reverse pose, bend right knee, and straighten left leg. Tighten left thigh muscles, and flex left foot. After stretching both legs, lean back in chair and relax.

☐ This gentle calf and hamstring stretch can be performed at home or at the office during a break from work.

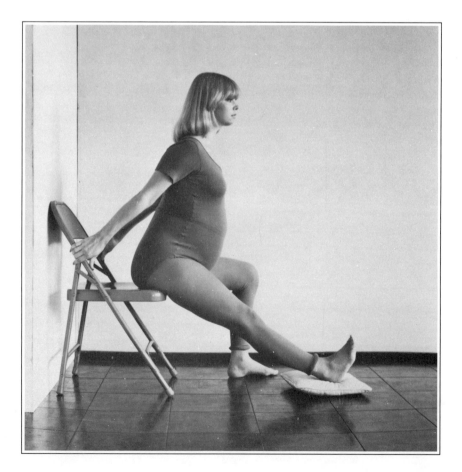

# Hamstring Stretch
# With Heel On Chair

☐ Place chair to wall. Pad chair with small pillow. Stand facing chair with feet parallel to each other.

☐ Bend left knee, raise leg, place heel on chair seat pillow, and straighten leg. Position right leg directly under right hip. Stand upright with hands on hips.

☐ Inhale and lift chest. Exhale and bend forward from hips keeping back straight. Tighten front thigh muscles and straighten both legs. Stretch should be felt in back of left thigh. If possible, extend arms and place hands high up on wall. Elongate spine with each exhalation.

☐ Remove left leg from chair and reverse. Place right heel on chair seat, left leg on floor, and bend forward from hips. Release pose and stand upright with arms at sides.

☐ This pose stretches hamstring and calf muscles.

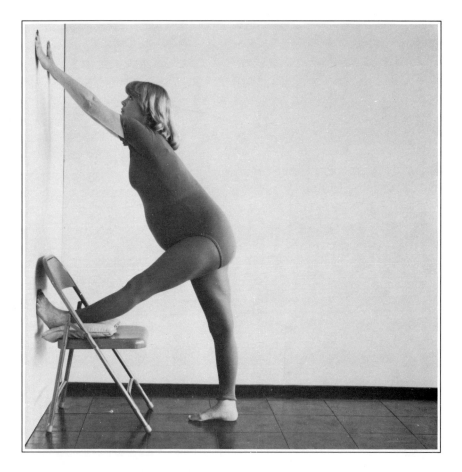

# Seated Alternate Leg Stretch To Wall

☐ Sit on mat or rug with back to wall and legs outstretched. Bend right knee and place sole of right foot against inner left thigh or left knee.

☐ Place hands beside hips. Push backwards until tailbone touches wall. Extend and straighten left leg on mat. Place strap around ball of left foot. Hold strap with both hands.

☐ Inhale, lift chest, and press entire back against wall. Exhale, pull back on strap, tighten front thigh muscles, and flex left foot. Concentrate on elongating spine up wall while stretching back of left leg.

☐ To reverse pose, bend left knee, and extend right leg. After stretching both legs, relax with back to wall.

☐ This pose stretches hamstring and calf muscles.

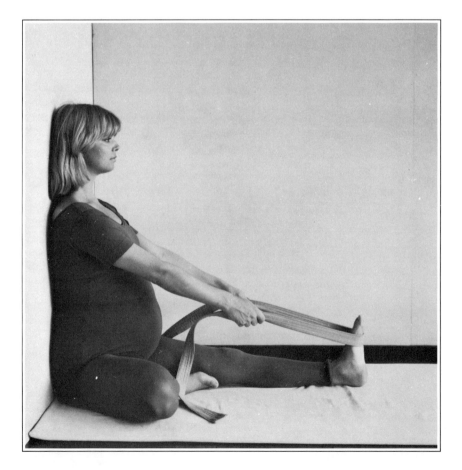

# Seated Alternate Leg Stretch With Chair

- [ ] Sit on mat in front of chair. Elevate buttocks with pillows or rolled blanket. Extend left leg under front chair rung.

- [ ] Bend right knee and place sole of right foot against inner left thigh or knee. Hold sides of chair and draw chair closer until sole of left foot touches back rung of chair. Tighten left front thigh muscles.

- [ ] Inhale, straighten arms, lift chest, and elongate spine. Exhale, extend heel under chair rung, and draw left toes toward knee. To increase hamstring stretch, bend forward from hips and reach higher up on chair back.

- [ ] To reverse pose, bend left knee, and extend right leg. After stretching both legs, cross legs and relax.

- [ ] This pose strengthens back muscles and stretches legs.

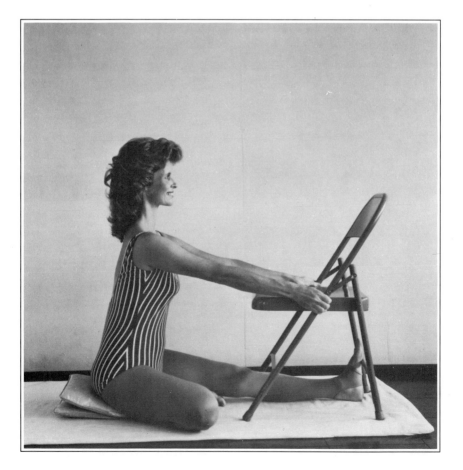

# Seated Alternate Leg Stretch

☐ Sit on mat or rug with legs outstretched. Elevate buttocks with pillow if necessary. Bend right knee and place sole of right foot against inner left thigh.

☐ Extend and straighten left leg on mat. Place strap around ball of left foot. Hold strap with both hands.

☐ Inhale, lift chest, and elongate spine. Exhale, pull back on strap, extend heel, and bend forward from hips. While stretching torso forward, maintain normal curves of spine. If necessary move hands down strap closer to foot.

☐ To reverse pose, bend left knee, and extend right leg. After stretching both legs, rest in a cross-legged position.

☐ This pose strengthens back muscles and stretches calf and hamstring muscles.

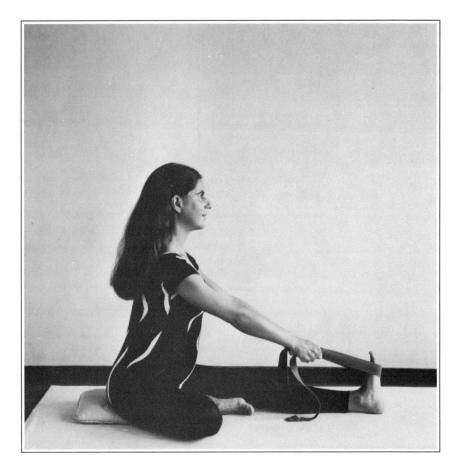

# Standing Hamstring Stretch To Wall

- ☐ Stand with back to wall. With heels 6 inches from wall, separate parallel feet 10-12 inches.

- ☐ Bend forward from hips and place strap under soles of feet. Straighten both legs, stretch buttock bones toward ceiling, and tighten front thigh muscles.

- ☐ Inhale, pull up on strap with both hands, and straighten elbows. Exhale, push buttock bones to wall, stretch chest forward, and elongate spine. Maintain normal spinal curves and rotate pelvis to bend forward.

- ☐ When spine is lengthened, release strap, bend knees, press lower back to wall, and relax leaning on wall.

- ☐ This pose relieves heaviness of uterus, stretches hamstring muscles evenly, and strengthens back muscles.

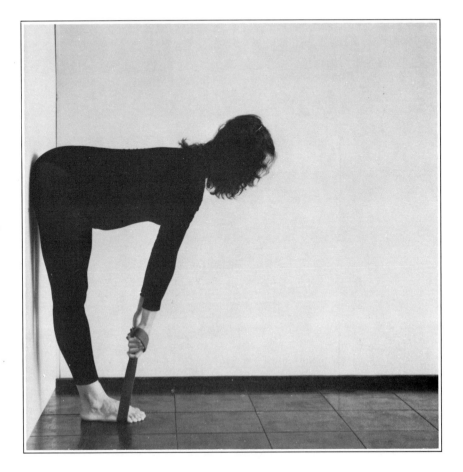

# Seated Hamstring Stretch

☐ Sit on rug or mat with both legs extended. Elevate buttocks with pillow. Feet may be separated.

☐ Place strap around balls of both feet. Hold strap evenly with both hands. Sit upright and look straight ahead.

☐ Inhale, lift top chest, and elongate spine. Exhale, pull back on strap, extend heels, and bend forward from hips. While stretching torso forward, maintain length of spine. If necessary move hands down strap closer to feet.

☐ With each exhalation entire upper body rotates forward over hip joints. Feet may separate to accomodate growing uterus. To release, bend knees, sit in comfortable cross-legged position, and relax.

☐ This position stretches hamstrings and strengthens back.

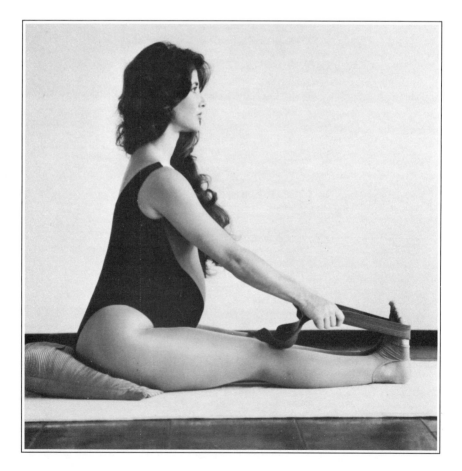

# Seated Hamstring Stretch With Chair

- [ ] Sit on mat in front of chair. Elevate buttocks with small pillows or rolled blanket.

- [ ] Extend both legs under front chair rung. Hold sides of chair and draw chair closer until soles of feet touch back rung of chair. If necessary for comfort, separate feet a few inches apart.

- [ ] Inhale, straighten arms, lift chest, and elongate spine. Exhale, extend heels, and draw toes toward knees. To increase stretch in hamstrings, bend forward from hips and hold back of seat or reach higher up on chair.

- [ ] To release, bend knees, sit in a comfortable cross-legged pose, and rest forehead on pillows placed on chair seat.

- [ ] This pose strengthens back and stretches hamstrings.

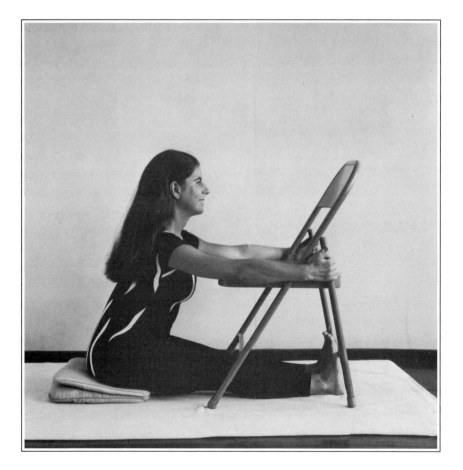

# Seated Wide Leg Stretch To Wall

☐ Sit on pillow or folded blanket facing wall. Widen legs and extend heels to wall. Place hands on floor behind hips, press down, elongate spine vertically, and stretch legs sideways. Keep knees and toes facing upward.

☐ Place hands high up on wall. Press legs down, lift top chest and sides of body, and bend forward at hips. With each exhalation, extend spine and relax shoulders. Widen legs if pose becomes too easy. Press backs of knees firmly to floor.

☐ To release, place hands on floor, ease away from wall, and rest in a comfortable cross-legged position with back to wall.

☐ This pose stretches inner thigh muscles and increases circulation in pelvic region.

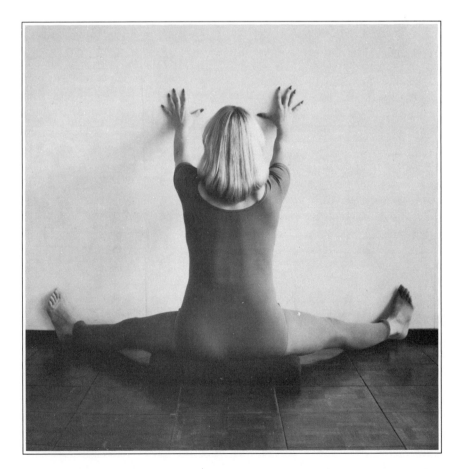

# Seated Wide Leg Stretch With Chair

☐ Sit on small pillow on floor in front of chair. Widen legs and place chair between legs a comfortable distance from abdomen. Rest forearms on chair seat.

☐ Press legs firmly into floor and extend heels. With each exhalation, press down with forearms, lift chest and stretch spine vertically.

☐ Close eyes, relax face muscles, and breathe slowly and evenly. For further relaxation, place a pile of pillows on chair seat, move chair slightly backward, bend forward, and rest forehead and folded arms on pillows.

☐ To release, move chair, and sit in a comfortable position.

☐ This posture provides a gentle inner leg stretch. It is especially appropriate during the third trimester.

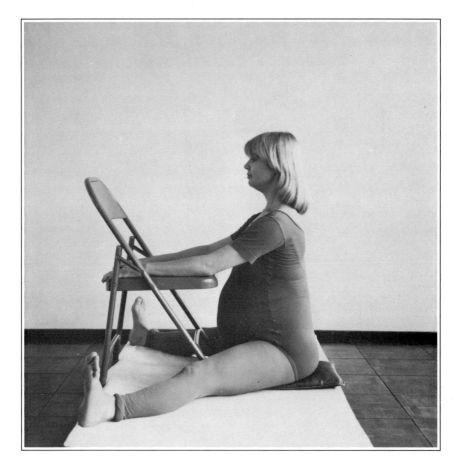

# Wide Leg Stretch

- [ ] Sit on folded blanket or pillow. Widen legs sideways, extend heels, lift kneecaps, and tighten front thigh muscles.

- [ ] Place hands on floor alongside hips. Press down with fingers, raise chest, and actively extend legs.

- [ ] Concentrate on expanding chest with each breath. If stretch becomes too easy, gradually widen legs. Keep backs of knees pressed firmly to floor.

- [ ] To release, place hands behind back, ease hips backward, bend knees, and gently bring legs together. Rest in a comfortable cross-legged sitting position.

- [ ] This posture stretches inner thigh muscles and lifts and expands chest.

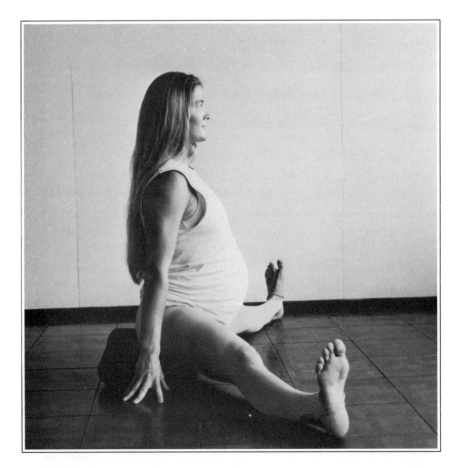

# Wide Leg Stretch
# With Forward Bend

☐ Sit on rug or mat. Widen legs sideways, extend heels, lift kneecaps, and contract front thigh muscles. Press legs firmly down into mat, and stretch toes upward.

☐ Lift sides of body and rotate forward at hips. Move spine as one unit by tilting top front pelvis forward. Legs remain firm as pelvis rotates forward in hip sockets.

☐ Stretch arms forward on floor. Press down with palms and extend breastbone forward. Use straight arms to control forward movement. With each exhalation stretch legs and elongate spine.

☐ To release, sit upright, and gently bring legs together.

☐ This pose stretches leg muscles and increases mobility of hip joints.

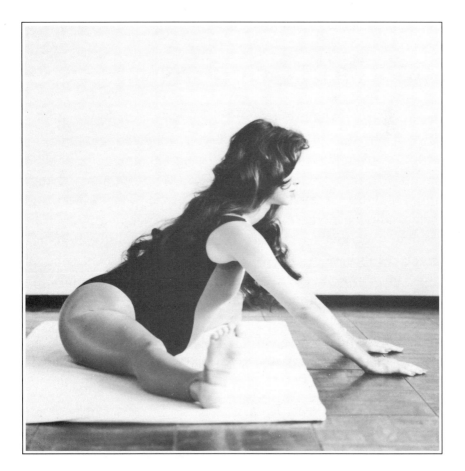

# Chapter 7

# THE TWISTING POSES

Twisting poses relieve a feeling of stiffness in the back. Gently twisting the torso massages the muscles along the spine and may help realign the vertebrae. Rotating the spine stimulates the nerves along the spinal column. With consistent practice, these postures may increase the ability of the spine to revolve.

Twisting poses also stretch the muscles of the neck, chest, back, and outer hips. Stretching these areas by twisting creates a feeling of freedom in the upper body. Releasing tight muscles may help alleviate back pain and reduce neck tension.

The depth of the inhalation of the breath depends on the ability of the rib cage to expand. Twisting poses also stretch the muscles of the rib cage and shoulder area. Stretching these muscles allows for greater expansion of the chest. This makes deeper breathing possible.

# Hints And Cautions

For maximum effectiveness, it is necessary to lengthen the spine while turning. If the spine is not elongated, the twist will be uneven. Coordinate the twisting movement with the breath. Lift the spine on an inhalation, and turn on an exhalation. Hold, take a few normal breaths in the new position, and then gradually increase the twist. Check to see that both shoulders are level. Allow the head to turn naturally. Forcing the head to rotate too far will strain the neck muscles.

During pregnancy twists should be performed gently to prevent overstretching. The majority of the twist will come from the neck, upper back, and shoulders. The neck can rotate approximately 45 to 50 degrees, and the upper back about 35 degrees. The lower back, designed mainly for side bending and forward and backward movement, is capable of only about 5 degrees of rotation.

The most vulnerable area is the *sacroiliac joint,* the joint where the sacrum joins the hip bone. This joint is designed for support, and it is supposed to remain stable. The sacroiliac joint is connected by strong ligaments. During pregnancy, the hormone relaxin loosens these ligaments. If twists are done forcibly, the sacroiliac joint may become unstable. This can happen on either side of the sacrum and may cause pain.

# Twisting Pose
# With Chair

☐ Sit sideways on chair seat with outer right thigh facing chair back. Place feet flat on floor and press knees together. Thighs and shins form a right angle. Rest hands on thighs and look straight ahead.

☐ Inhale, squeeze legs together, lift chest, and lengthen spine vertically. While exhaling, hold sides of chair back and twist torso toward right. Breathe normally and gradually increase twist. Shoulders will twist the most and lower back will twist the least.

☐ Change sides. Sit with left thigh facing chair back. Hold sides of chair back and gently twist toward left. After twisting to both sides, lean back in chair and relax.

☐ This pose stretches shoulder muscles and massages back muscles.

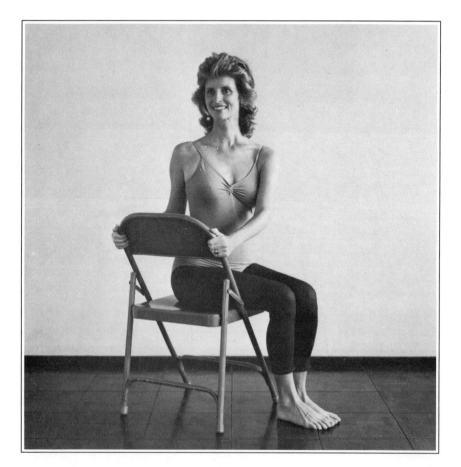

# Revolved Foot To Thigh Pose

- [ ] Sit on mat or rug and separate legs sideways. Bend left knee and place left foot to inside of right thigh.

- [ ] Place hands beside hips, press down to lift spine, extend and straighten right leg, and flex right foot.

- [ ] Inhale, hold outer left thigh with right hand, and place left hand on floor behind back. Exhale, lift spine vertically, and gently twist toward left.

- [ ] To reverse, change legs. Bend right knee and place right foot to inner left thigh. Hold right thigh with left hand, place right hand on floor, and twist toward right.

- [ ] After twisting to both sides, bend knees, and sit in a comfortable cross-legged position with spine straight.

- [ ] This pose increases lateral rotation of spine.

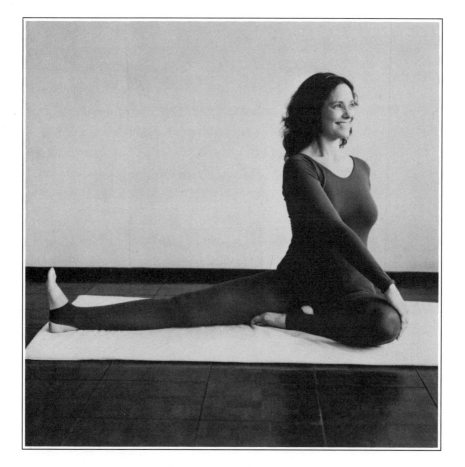

# Knee To Wall
# Twist

☐ Sit on floor or rug next to wall. Place outer left leg against wall and extend both legs straight ahead. Bend left knee, press outer thigh to wall, and position left foot flat on floor. Bend left elbow and place left upper arm or elbow to inner thigh of left leg on wall.

☐ Tighten front thigh muscles of right leg. Extend right heel and draw toes toward right knee.

☐ Inhale, lift chest and lengthen spine. Exhale, press left knee to wall, gently twist toward right, and place right hand on floor. Head and shoulders may rest on wall.

☐ To reverse, change sides. Bend right knee and press to wall, extend left leg, and twist to left. Release and rest.

☐ This pose massages back and shoulder muscles.

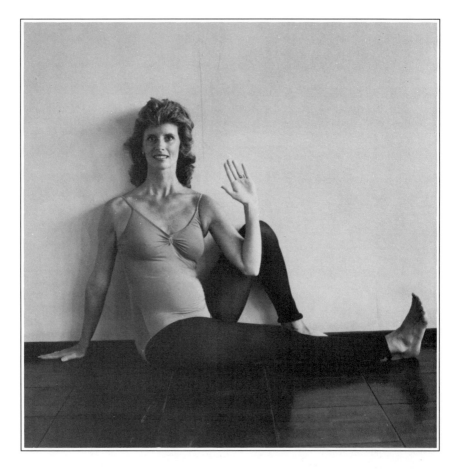

# Wide Leg Stretch
# With Twist

- [ ] Sit on mat or rug. Widen legs sideways, extend heels, tighten front thigh muscles, and press backs of knees to floor. Toes and kneecaps face ceiling. Place hands on floor alongside hips. Press down with fingers, elongate spine, and actively extend legs.

- [ ] To gently twist toward right, place left hand on floor in line with navel and right hand on floor behind right hip. With an exhalation lift chest and twist toward right.

- [ ] Place both hands on floor behind hips, move torso to center, and rest. Move right hand to floor in line with navel, exhale, and gradually twist toward left.

- [ ] To release, place hands behind back, ease hips backward, bend knees, carefully bring legs together, and relax.

- [ ] This pose stretches inner thigh and spinal muscles.

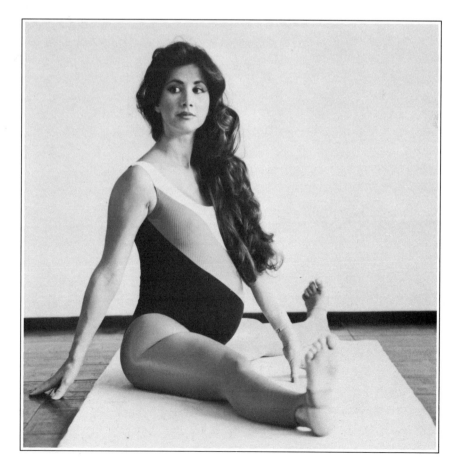

# Seated Bent Knee Twist

- [ ] Sit on mat or rug with legs outstretched. Bend both knees, fold lower legs back, and place feet beside right hip. Instep of right foot fits in arch of left foot. Separate knees slightly and lower right hip toward floor.

- [ ] Inhale, hold left outer thigh or knee with right hand, and place left hand on floor behind back. Exhale, lift chest, elongate spine, and gently twist shoulders to left. Turn head to left, or turn head and look over right shoulder.

- [ ] To twist to right, extend legs and reverse pose. Bend knees, place feet beside left hip, hold right knee, and gradually twist toward right. Release, extend legs, and rest in a comfortable cross-legged sitting position.

- [ ] This pose massages spinal muscles and stretches outer hip, shoulder, and neck muscles.

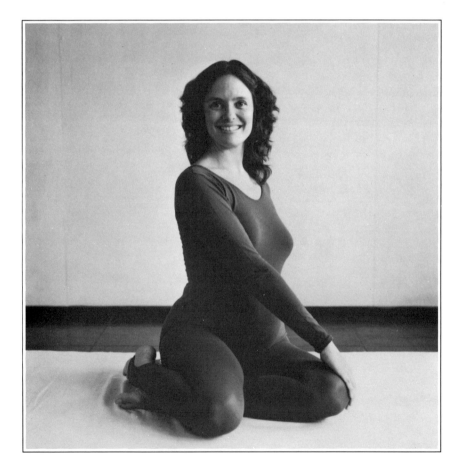

# Chapter 8

# THE BREATHING AWARENESS AND RELAXATION POSES

The ability to relax creates the confidence necessary to maintain a positive attitude throughout the birth process. As long as a pregnant woman can fully relax during contractions, she will be ready for the next one. Relaxation methods need to be learned early in pregnancy and practiced regularly. They can be applied effectively to potentially stressful situations arising during labor and birth.

The training involves establishing a close relationship between the body and the breath. This is called *breath awareness*, and it is nothing more than coordinating the exhalation of the breath with the movements of the body.

To learn this technique, sit on a pillow with the back against the wall, bend both knees, and place the soles of the feet together. Inhale and lift the spine. Exhale, close the eyes, and release the thighs toward the floor. Gradually soften the muscles of the inner thighs with each successive exhalation. Consistent practice of this pose will prove useful during the pushing stage of labor. When the coach or nurse asks for relaxation of the inner thighs, the response will be automatic.

Practicing passive relaxation in a side-lying position may relieve muscular tension and mental anxiety. This is done by quieting the mind and directing conscious attention to specific areas of the body. When a tense area is located, that area is gently encouraged to relax. This may be accomplished by a variety of means. The area can be actively tensed and then released, or the breath can be directed to the tense place. The tight area can be covered by an image of something soft or warm. The methods vary, but tension *can* be released through focused relaxation. After tight parts are let go, a deeper state of relaxation will naturally occur.

The above passive relaxation technique is particularly appropriate during the first stage of labor. Between contractions, tense areas can be identified and relaxed. With this release of tension, it may be possible to fall asleep between subsequent contractions. Relaxing during the early stage of labor will conserve energy for the active second stage, and the birth itself.

# Hints And Cautions

In order for total relaxation to occur, the body must feel balanced, safe, and supported. Practice the following poses in an airy, quiet place away from interruptions. Use plenty of pillows and blankets for comfort. When the body is at ease, the mind can begin to relax.

Every pregnant woman needs a daily period of quiet seclusion. During this time she can reflect on the constant changes occuring within her body. She can contemplate her attitudes toward pregnancy, her fears of inadequacy, and consider ways of increasing her confidence. Therefore, setting aside a time for daily reflection and relaxation is essential for the development of mental and physical well-being.

# Breathing Awareness Pose

☐ Sit on rug or mat. Bring soles of feet together or sit in any comfortable cross-legged pose. Rest back against partner's back or against wall. Relax hands on feet or thighs with palms up. Lift chest and elongate spine.

☐ Take a few normal breaths and allow eyes to close. Begin to gradually deepen breath. Take slow, deep, smooth inhalations and normal exhalations.

☐ With each inhalation open ribs sideways. While sitting back to back, synchronize breathing with partner's breathing, and feel breath expanding side and back ribs.

☐ At top of inhalation lift breastbone. Keep throat and face muscles relaxed. Exhale softly and naturally. To release, stretch out legs, and breathe normally.

☐ Breathing awareness is essential for relaxation in labor.

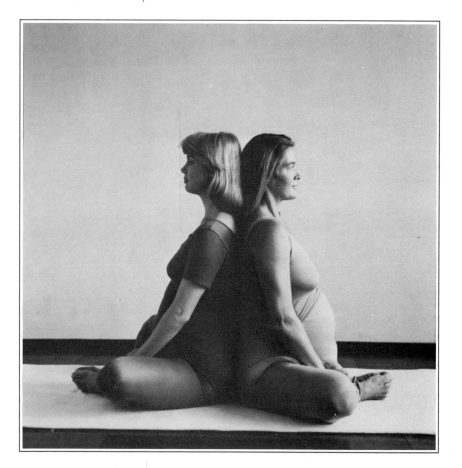

# Child's Pose

☐ Kneel on mat or blanket. Sit back on heels and widen knees. Bend at hips, stretch torso forward between legs, and rest forehead on mat or pillow.

☐ Press buttocks to heels and stretch arms straight forward to lengthen back. For deeper relaxation, rest arms alongside legs, or relax head on folded forearms.

☐ For lower back relief, have partner place palms on sacrum and gradually press down and back toward feet.

☐ Consciously relax entire spine and chest. Release tension in muscles with each exhalation. Remain in pose until whole body feels relaxed.

☐ This pose relieves lower back tension and teaches conscious relaxation.

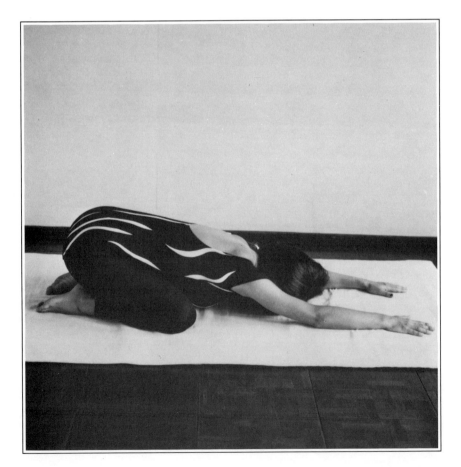

# Lower Back Relaxation Pose With Chair

- [ ] Place firm bolster or stack of blankets in front of chair. Sit sideways on bolster. Lower hands onto floor behind bolster. Lean on hands and swing legs onto chair seat.

- [ ] Lift and adjust hips until buttocks rest in center of bolster. Carefully lower spine toward floor. Shoulders and upper back will rest on mat.

- [ ] Relax arms at sides, or bend elbows and rest backs of hands and forearms on mat. Rest lower legs on chair seat.

- [ ] Close eyes and breathe slowly and deeply. Release jaw and facial muscles and allow spinal muscles to relax. To release, bend knees, slide hips off front edge of pillow, roll onto one side, and push up to sitting positon.

- [ ] This pose removes fatigue and reduces back tension.

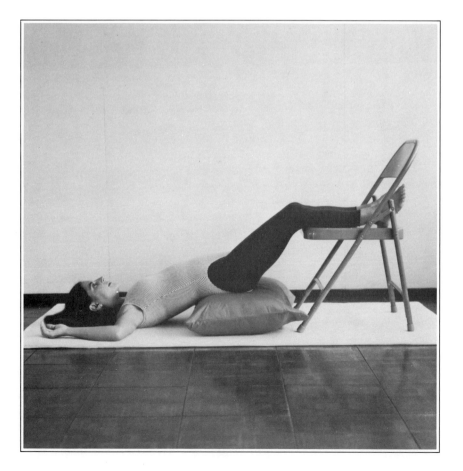

# Legs Up Wall
# Relaxation Pose

☐ Place firm bolster or stack of blankets 6 inches from wall. Sit sideways on bolster with right hip toward wall.

☐ Place left hand on floor and right hand on bolster. Lower spine onto bolster, turn hips toward right, and swing both legs up wall. Adjust hips and rest buttocks and lower back on bolster. Head and shoulders relax on mat.

☐ Relax arms beside bolster, or bend elbows and rest backs of hands and forearms on mat.

☐ Close eyes and relax completely. Breathe slowly and evenly, expanding ribs sideways with each inhalation. To release, place feet on wall, slide buttocks off pillow onto floor, roll onto one side, and sit up.

☐ This relaxing pose relieves leg and back fatigue. It naturally calms the mind without using any mental effort.

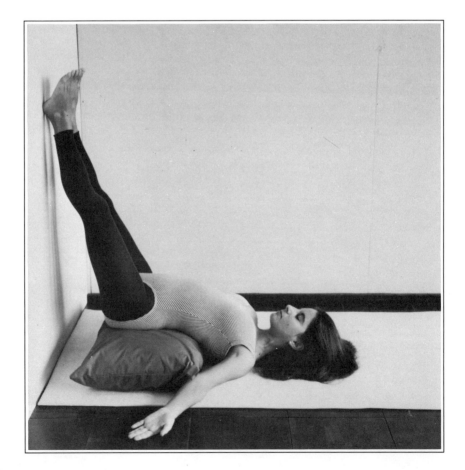

# Back-Lying Relaxation Pose

☐ Arrange a wedge-shaped pile of pillows on mat or rug. Sit on mat with legs outstretched. Place narrow end of pillow pile against tailbone.

☐ Lower spine onto pillows. Adjust pillows for comfort and balance. Elevate head and chest higher than hips. Forearms rest on mat with palms facing upward.

☐ Separate feet 8-12 inches apart. Release hips and allow legs to roll outward. Adjust body until left and right sides are symmetrical. Let body sink into mat and pillows.

☐ Consciously release tension in each part of body. Pay special attention to softening jaw and facial muscles. Breathe slowly and evenly, and allow body to relax. To release pose, bend knees, roll onto side, and sit up.

☐ This pose releases tension throughout entire body.

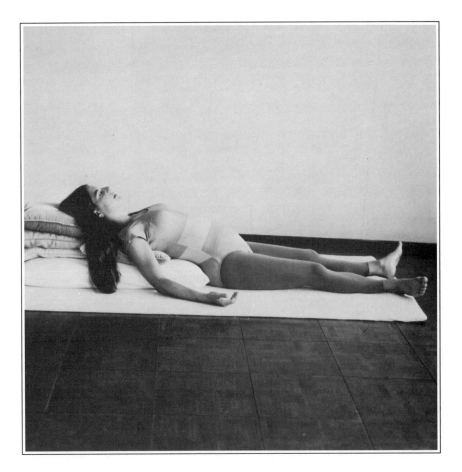

# Elevated Leg
# Side-Lying Pose

- [ ] Pad chair seat and place chair to wall. Place stack of blankets or firm bolster in front of chair. Lie on left side with left hip raised on bolster and left shoulder on mat.

- [ ] Bend left leg and elevate right lower leg on chair seat. Adjust distance from chair for comfort. Support head and neck with pillows and relax arms.

- [ ] Consciously release tension in muscles and joints. Breathe gently and evenly. When fatigue in right leg is lessened, remove leg from chair and change sides. Lie on right side and elevate left leg.

- [ ] To release pose, remove left leg from chair, push up to a sitting position, and relax.

- [ ] This pose removes fatigue in legs and swelling in ankles.

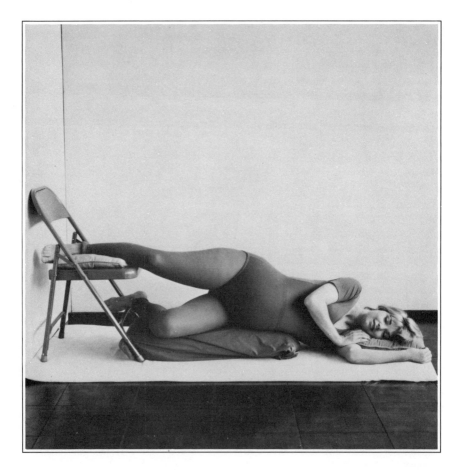

# Side-Lying Relaxation Pose

☐ Lie on left side on mat or rug. Support head and neck with pillows. Adjust left shoulder for comfort. Elevate right knee with pillows. Relax fingers completely.

☐ Systematically relax all muscles and joints in body. Begin by releasing foot, calf, and thigh muscles. Soften ankle, knee, and hip joints. Allow legs to feel heavy and sink into mat and pillows.

☐ Breathe into base of spine. Feel entire spine softening and relaxing. Let go of tension in neck and shoulder joints. Imagine tiredness flowing out of fingertips.

☐ Relax jaw and soften facial muscles. Close eyes, separate lips slightly, and breathe normally. When tension is released, slowly push up to a sitting position.

☐ This pose creates complete relaxation of body and mind.

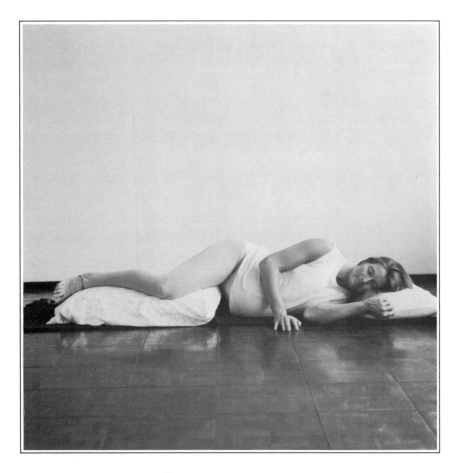

# Chapter 9

# THE POSTNATAL POSES

All the poses in the previous chapters can be practiced after the baby is born. The additional postures introduced in this chapter concentrate on strengthening the abdominal muscles which were overstretched during pregnancy.

This section also includes twists which help shrink the uterus. Relaxation poses are added to lessen fatigue and aid in the recovery from childbirth.

All the poses are illustrated with the baby nearby. It is not necessary to do the poses with your baby, but it may be a very pleasant experience. Many women find it difficult to find time to exercise after the baby is born. In order to be with the baby when he or she is awake, mothers usually do household tasks when the baby is asleep. Therefore, doing yoga postures with your baby will help you get back in shape while enjoying the company of your baby.

# Hints And Cautions

Do not be in a hurry to flatten your abdomen by beginning strenuous exercises right after childbirth. Regaining your original muscle tone takes time, and it is important to procede cautiously.

Strengthen the pelvic floor muscles first with vaginal contraction exercises. Alternately contract and relax the sphincter muscles around the opening to the vagina. These exercises increase circulation and will aid healing, restore lost sensation, and tighten vaginal muscles.

Back-lying pelvic tilting poses may be practiced in conjunction with the vaginal contraction exercises. With knees bent, exhale and press the lower back into the floor while contracting the vaginal muscles. This will begin to strengthen stretched abdominal muscles.

The abdominal muscles are in a weakened state, and need to be gradually and consistently strengthened. A *hernia*, or rupture caused by the separation of the rectus muscles of the abdomen, can occur during pregnancy or childbirth. If you notice a small bulge in the abdomen, do not attempt abdominal strengthening poses, and inform your physician.

The back muscles are sensitive after birth and can be easily overstrained. The ligaments are softened by relaxin, and the sacroiliac joint may be unstable. To protect the spine, do abdominal tightening exercises in a back-lying position.

After a Caesarean birth, it is necessary to wait six weeks before beginning a regular exercise program. Three weeks wait is sufficient after a vaginal birth.

Begin with the seated forward bending poses covered in Chapter 6. Place loosely rolled blankets on your thighs, relax forward, and rest the chest and forehead on the blankets. Twisting poses are the next group of poses to add. The twists in this chapter can be supplemented with those in Chapter 7. Both twists and forward bends massage the uterus. This massage helps the uterus return to its normal size.

When energy begins to return, performing the standing poses in Chapter 3 will help regain lost leg strength and endurance. The abdominal strengthening poses in this chapter may be added next.

The shoulder stretches in Chapter 2 will help relieve the neck and shoulder tension caused by nursing and carrying your baby. While nursing your baby, use pillows for support, and arrange yourself in a balanced, comfortable position.

Inverted poses, such as the shoulderstand pose with a chair, are added last. They should be postponed until the *lochia*, the postpartum discharge from the uterus, has ceased.

Taking time for a daily period of reflection and relaxation can be an invaluable aid in adjusting to the demands of new motherhood. Relaxation poses can renew lost energy and may be enjoyed with the sleeping baby.

# Knee To Chest
# Lower Back Stretch

- ☐ Lie on mat or rug. Place small pillow under head. Baby may lie on blanket beside you.

- ☐ Bend knees and lift thighs toward chest. Interlace fingers below front of knees.

- ☐ Inhale and expand chest. Exhale, press lower back to mat, and pull knees toward chest. Massage muscles on either side of spine by gently rolling from side to side.

- ☐ Bring knees slowly toward chest to gradually stretch lower back muscles. Lift forehead toward chest to stretch and strengthen neck muscles.

- ☐ To release, lower arms, roll onto one side, and sit up.

- ☐ This pose releases tension in lower back.

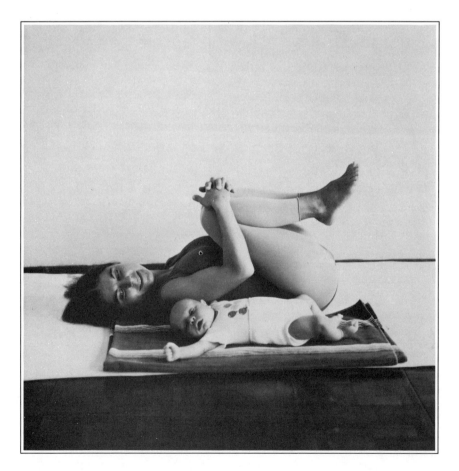

# Elbow To Opposite Knee Curl-Up

☐ Lie on back on mat or rug. Place baby on blanket alongside you. Extend legs on floor.

☐ Inhale and interlace fingers behind head. Exhale, lift head and shoulders off mat, bring left elbow toward right knee, and extend left leg. Press back of head lightly. Roll down and relax. Repeat to other side. Curl up and bring right elbow toward bent left knee. Release and relax.

☐ For an easier variation of pose, begin with both knees bent, feet on floor, and arms alongside body. On an exhalation press lower back to floor, curl head and shoulders off mat, and stretch both arms to outside of right knee. Roll down and relax. Repeat pose to other side. Release, roll over onto one side, and sit up.

☐ This pose strengthens oblique abdominal muscles.

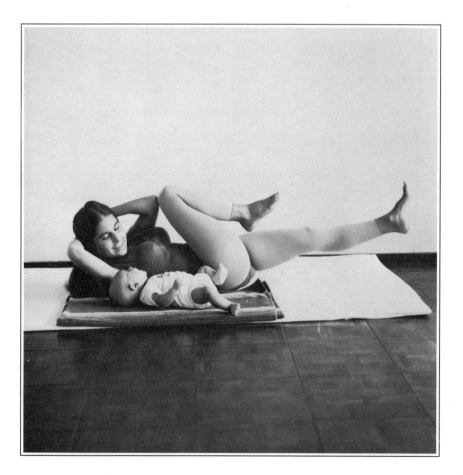

# Curl-Ups With Feet On Wall

Post

- ☐ Lie on back on mat with knees bent and feet to wall. Baby may be on blanket beside you, or resting on thighs.

- ☐ Lift legs and place feet flat on wall. Shins are parallel to floor. Inhale and relax, exhale and press lower back firmly to floor.

- ☐ Keep lower back on floor and inhale. Exhale and slowly curl head, shoulders, and upper back off floor. On next exhalation, roll spine down, and relax. Repeat 2 times. When strength permits, gradually build up to 10 curl-ups.

- ☐ To release, place baby on blanket, bend knees, roll onto one side, and push up to a comfortable sitting position.

- ☐ Curl-ups help tone abdomen after childbirth by strengthening abdominal muscles.

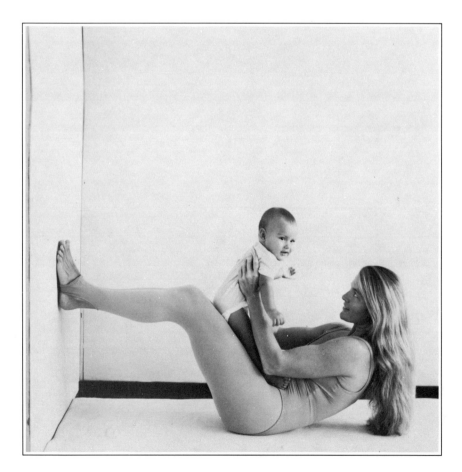

# Bridge Pose
# With Baby

- ☐ Lie on back on mat or rug. Place baby on abdomen or alongside you on blanket.

- ☐ Bend knees and place feet flat on floor. Place feet parallel to each other and 6-8 inches apart.

- ☐ Inhale and relax back. Exhale and flatten lower back to floor. On next exhalation press down with feet, lift hips off floor, and curl tailbone upward. Lift pelvis higher than abdomen and squeeze knees together. Lower spine to floor and relax. Repeat pose twice.

- ☐ To release pose, place baby on blanket, bend knees, roll onto one side, and push up to a sitting position.

- ☐ This pose strengthens knees, buttocks, and abdominal muscles, and may alleviate back tension.

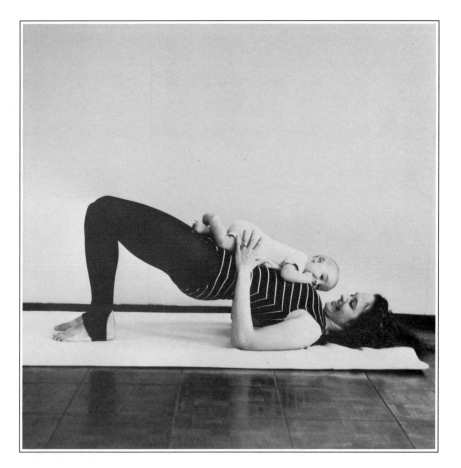

# Shoulderstand
# With Chair

☐ Begin pose 4-6 weeks after birth. Place chair to wall. Arrange 2 inch high stack of folded blankets in front of chair on mat. Lie on back with knees bent. Align shoulders with edge of blankets. Back of head rests on floor and arms rest at sides. Baby may lie beside you.

☐ With back resting on blankets, lift legs one at a time and place parallel feet flat on chair seat. Inhale, press down with feet and arms. Exhale, lift hips upward, move chest toward chin, extend arms, and hold front legs of chair.

☐ Breathe normally and tuck tailbone. Move top front pelvis toward navel and lengthen lower back. Hold for 1-2 minutes and lower back onto floor. To release, bend knees, roll onto one side, and sit up. This pose opens chest, stretches shoulders and neck, and tightens buttocks and back thigh muscles.

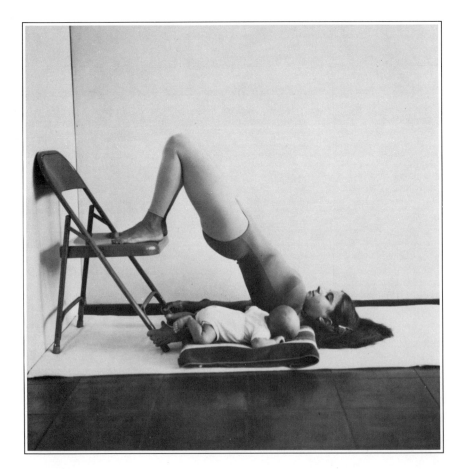

# Standing Hamstring Stretch With Chair

- [ ] Place chair to wall. Pad chair seat with pillows. Baby may rest on blankets beside chair or be held during pose.

- [ ] Hold baby and stand in front of chair. Bend left knee, place heel on chair seat pillow, and straighten leg. Align right leg directly under right hip. Extend left heel and tighten front thigh muscles. Support baby on left thigh.

- [ ] Inhale and lift chest. Exhale and bend slightly forward from hips. Maintain normal curves of spine. Stretch will be felt in back of left thigh and calf.

- [ ] To change sides, remove baby from thigh, bend left knee and stand with feet together. Bend right knee, place right heel on chair, and bend forward from hips. Release pose.

- [ ] This pose develops leg strength, and stretches hamstring and calf muscles.

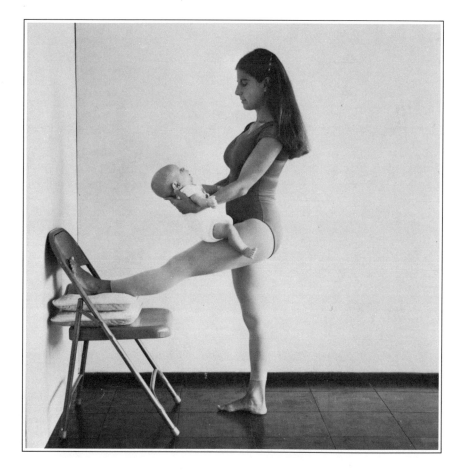

# Elevated Downward Dog Pose

☐ Place bench, blocks, or stack of books to wall. Pose may also be performed on lower step of staircase. Lay baby on blanket in front of bench. Place palms 8-10 inches apart on top of bench.

☐ Straighten arms and walk feet well back. Position parallel feet 8-12 inches apart. Tighten front thigh muscles, completely straighten legs, and lift buttock bones toward ceiling. Relax neck muscles.

☐ Inhale and push down on bench to stretch arms and shoulders. Exhale and lengthen entire back away from hands. Breathe normally and descend head and chest.

☐ When back is fully extended, release, and stand upright.

☐ This pose relieves lower back tension and stretches hamstring, shoulder, and spinal muscles.

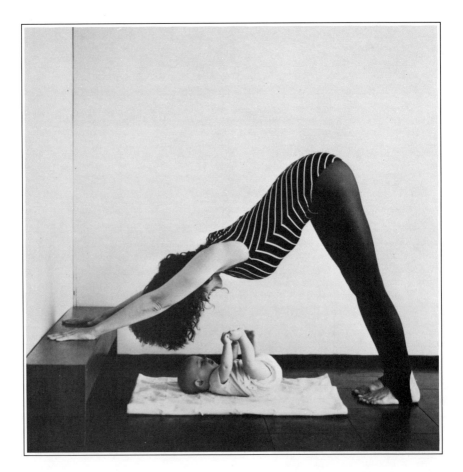

# Seated Twist On Bench Or Chair

Post

☐ Place bench or chair to wall. Pose may also be performed sitting on steps of a staircase.

☐ Lay baby on blanket in front of bench or staircase. With knees and feet together sit on front edge of bench, step, or chair. Position elbow and back of upper left arm to outer right thigh. Place right hand on bench, step, or wall.

☐ Inhale, squeeze knees together, and lift chest. Exhale, press left elbow to right thigh, and twist torso toward right. Elongate spine with each exhalation. Change sides. Press right elbow to left thigh, and twist toward left.

☐ To release, stretch chest forward over thighs, and relax.

☐ This pose strengthens oblique abdominal muscles and helps uterus return to normal size.

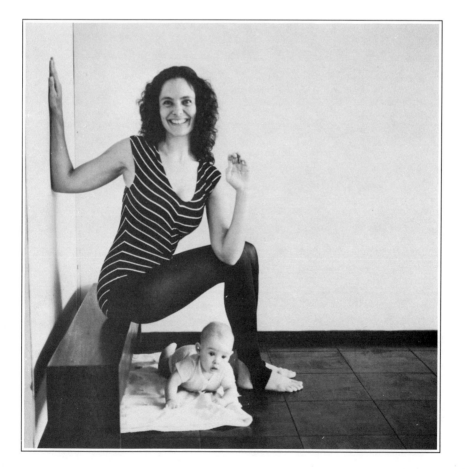

# Kneeling Twist To Wall

- [ ] Kneel 1 to 1 1/2 feet from wall. Lay baby on blanket beside you. Lower buttocks onto heels.

- [ ] Position right elbow to outside of left thigh. Inhale and lengthen spine. Exhale, press right elbow against left knee, and twist torso toward left. Bend left elbow and place left hand on wall to aid rotation of spine in twist.

- [ ] Change sides. Press left elbow against right knee, and twist torso toward right. Bend right elbow and place right hand on wall to increase twist.

- [ ] To release, remove hand from wall, separate knees slightly, and stretch torso forward between legs. Relax forehead on floor. Release and sit upright.

- [ ] This pose helps align spinal vertebrae, massages back muscles, and stretches outer hip muscles.

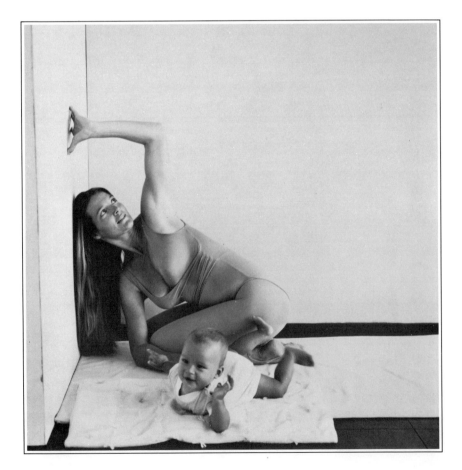

# Reclining Foot On Thigh Twist

( Post )

☐ Lie on back on mat or rug with legs extended. Support head with small pillow if desired. Place baby beside you. Bend left knee. Place left foot on front of right thigh. Right leg on mat may be straight or slightly bent.

☐ Inhale, expand chest, and hold left knee with right hand. Exhale, twist hips to right and press knee toward floor. Extend left arm on mat, roll left shoulder toward floor, turn head, and look over left arm. Breathe normally.

☐ Change sides. Bend right knee, place right foot on left thigh, and press right knee toward floor. Legs move toward left. Spine, shoulders, and head twist toward right.

☐ To release, bend both knees toward chest, roll over onto one side, and push up to a sitting position.

☐ This pose stretches outer hip, back, and shoulder muscles.

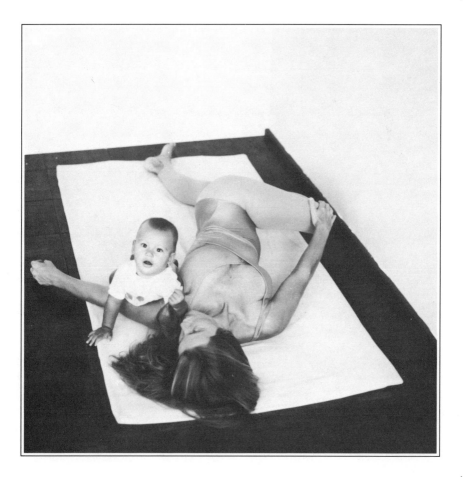

# Pelvic Tilt Relaxation Pose With Chair

- ☐ Place chair on mat. Lie down on back in front of chair. Baby may rest on abdomen. Extra weight of baby on mother's abdomen relaxes back. Bend knees and rest lower legs on chair seat. Relax head, upper arms, and back on mat.

- ☐ Inhale and expand chest. Exhale and press lower back firmly into mat. With each exhalation lengthen lower back muscles by flattening back on mat.

- ☐ If baby is asleep, close your eyes and rest. Release jaw and facial muscles and allow lower back to relax.

- ☐ To release, place baby on mat, remove legs from chair, bend knees toward chest, roll onto one side, and sit up.

- ☐ This pose removes leg fatigue and reduces back tension.

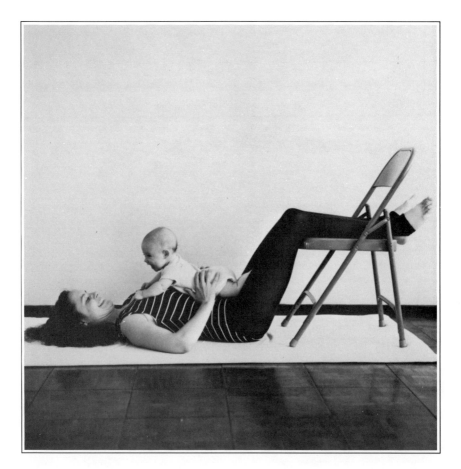

# Chest Opening Relaxation Pose

☐ Place firm bolster or stack of blankets to wall. Sit sideways on bolster with right hip against wall.

☐ Place left hand on floor and right hand on bolster. Lower spine onto bolster, turn hips toward right, and swing both legs up wall. Adjust hips, and rest buttocks and lower back on bolster. Head and shoulders relax on mat.

☐ Hold baby on abdomen or lay baby beside you. Either press buttocks and backs of legs to wall, or move hips slightly away from wall.

☐ If baby is asleep, close eyes and relax completely for 5 to 10 minutes. To release, lay baby on mat, place feet on wall, slide buttocks off bolster, roll onto side, and sit up.

☐ This relaxing pose relieves leg and back fatigue, and removes shoulder tension created by nursing.

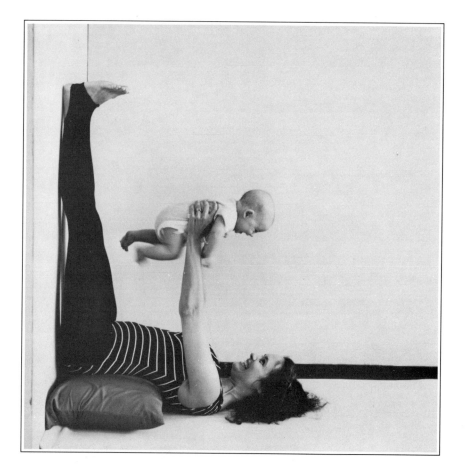

# Reclining Wide Leg Pose To Wall

☐ Lie on mat or rug with buttocks touching wall and legs up wall. Widen legs sideways, press backs of knees to wall, and extend heels. Relax inner thighs.

☐ Place baby on abdomen or on mat beside you. Completely relax back, shoulders, upper arms, and head on mat. If desired, add a small pillow behind head.

☐ If baby is asleep, close your eyes and completely relax. Breathe slowly and smoothly, expanding rib cage sideways with each inhalation. Relax facial muscles.

☐ Remain in pose 5 to 10 minutes. To release, lay baby beside you, slowly bend knees toward chest, roll onto one side, and sit up with back resting against wall.

☐ This relaxing pose stretches inner leg muscles.

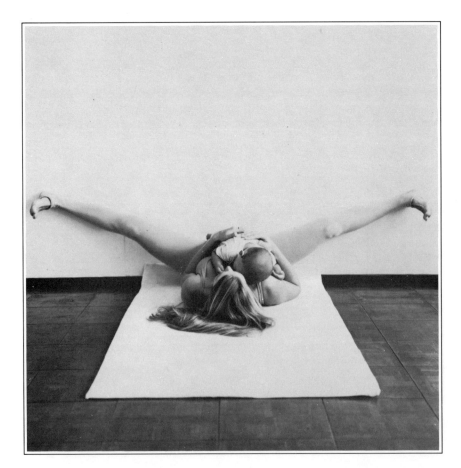

# Reclining Bound Angle Pose

☐ Lie on back on mat with buttocks touching wall and legs extended up wall. Lay baby on abdomen or place on mat beside you.

☐ Widen legs sideways, bend knees, and place soles of feet together. Allow heels to descend toward pelvic floor. For additional inner thigh stretch, press thighs to wall.

☐ If baby is sleeping, close your eyes and relax. With each exhalation release inner thighs, spine, and facial muscles. Rest arms at sides and breathe normally.

☐ Remain in pose 5 minutes. To release, place baby beside you, lift legs, bring knees together, roll onto one side, and sit up with back resting on wall.

☐ This pose relaxes back and stretches inner thigh muscles.

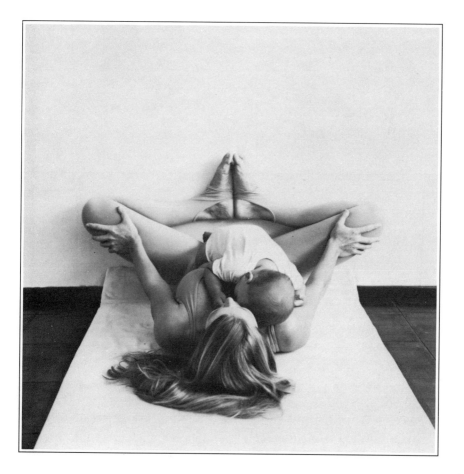

# Sample Program
# For First Trimester

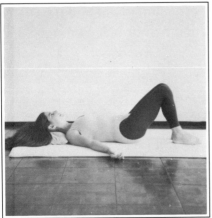

Reclining Pelvic Tilt (p. 10)

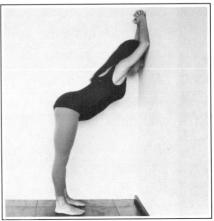

Forearms on Wall Shoulder
Stretch (p. 17)

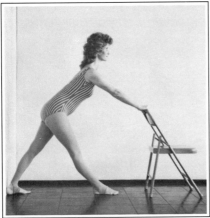

Alternate Leg Stretch with Chair
(p. 30)

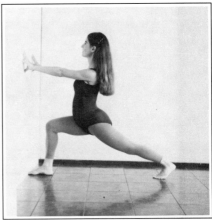

Warrior I Pose to Wall (p. 39)

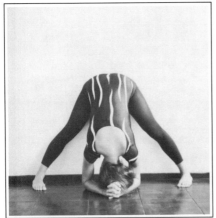

Head to Floor Wide Leg Stretch
(p. 41)

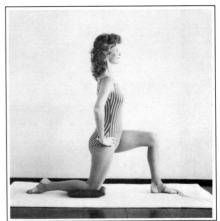

Kneeling Front Thigh Stretch
(p.50)

The following 12 poses are appropriate during the first three months of pregnancy. For instructions, refer to the page number listed after the title. Practice back-lying poses only in the first trimester.

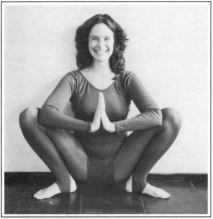

Squatting Pose to Wall (p. 58)

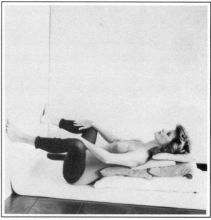

Hip Stretch with Feet on Wall (p. 60)

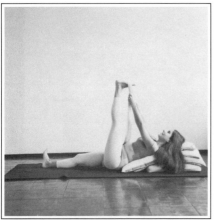

Reclining Alternate Leg Hamstring Stretch (p. 68)

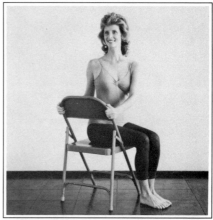

Twisting Pose with Chair (p. 84)

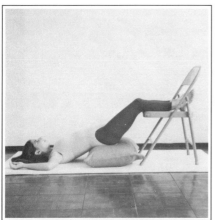

Lower Back Relaxation Pose with Chair (p. 93)

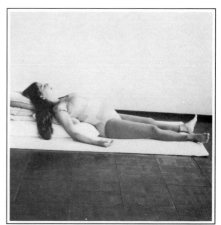

Back-Lying Relaxation Pose (p. 95)

# Sample Program
# For Second Trimester

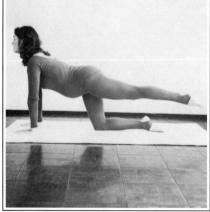

Cat Stretch with Leg Lift (p. 13)

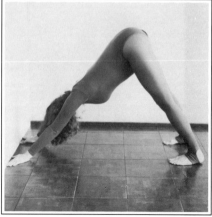

Downward Dog Pose (p. 24)

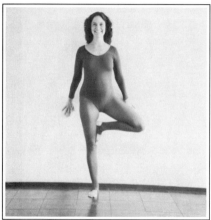

Tree Pose (p. 28)

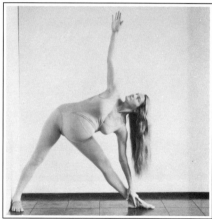

Triangle Pose (p. 32)

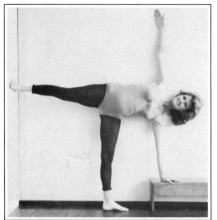

Half Moon Pose with Wall
(p. 38)

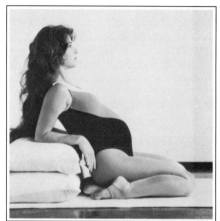

Half Reclining Hero's Pose
(p. 45)

The following 12 poses are appropriate for the second trimester of pregnancy. These poses concentrate on strengthening legs, and stretching hip, front thigh, and hamstring muscles.

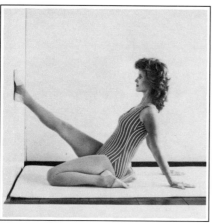

Elevated Leg and Front Thigh Stretch (p. 54)

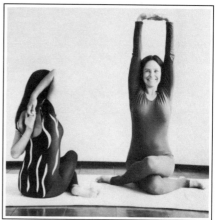

Shoulder Stretches in Leg Over Leg Pose (p. 64)

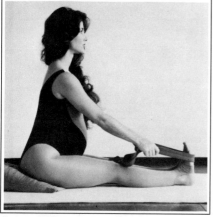

Seated Hamstring Stretch (p. 76)

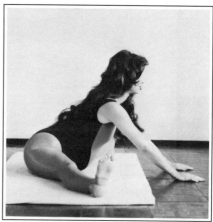

Wide Leg Stretch with Forward Bend (p. 81)

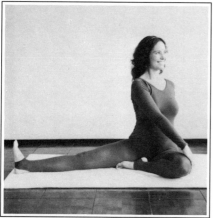

Revolved Foot to Thigh Pose (p. 85)

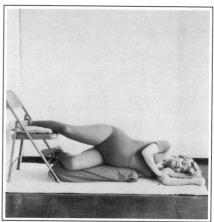

Elevated Leg Side-Lying Pose (p. 96)

# Sample Program
# For Third Trimester

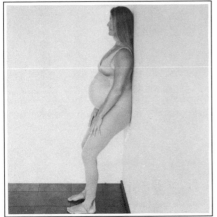

Basic Standing Posture (p. 9)

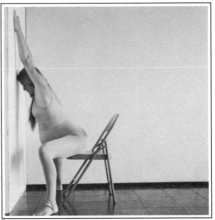

Seated Shoulder Stretch (p. 20)

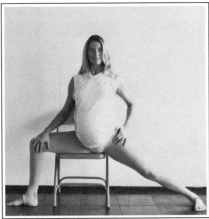

Warrior II Pose with Chair
(p. 34)

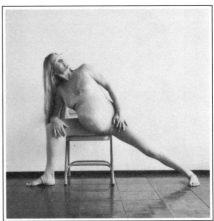

Side Angle Pose with Chair
(p. 37)

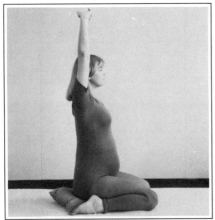

Hero's Pose with Arms Overhead (p. 44)

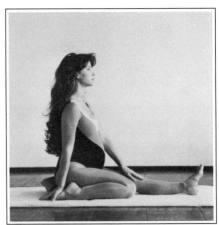

Seated Alternate Front Thigh
Stretch (p. 52)

The following 12 poses are suitable for the last three months of pregnancy. These poses concentrate on breathing, relaxation, and stretching with the support of a chair.

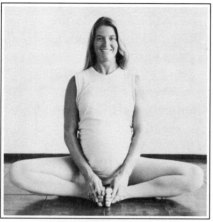

Bound Angle Pose (p. 59)

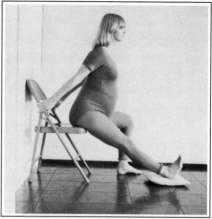

Easy Hamstring Stretch in Chair (p. 70)

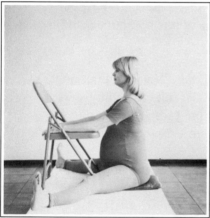

Seated Wide Leg Stretch with Chair (p. 79)

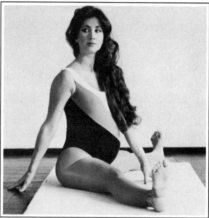

Wide Leg Stretch with Twist (p. 87)

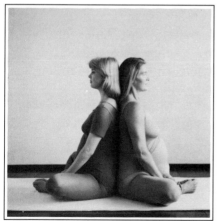

Breathing Awareness Pose (p. 91)

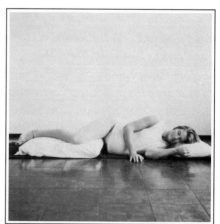

Side-Lying Relaxation Pose (p. 97)

# Recommended Reading

*Essential Exercises for the Childbearing Year* by Elizabeth Noble, R.P.T., Houghton Mifflin Company, Boston, Massachusetts, 1976. Detailed explanations of physical changes and problems during pregnancy. Concentrates on the pelvic floor, abdominal muscles, posture, relaxation, breathing, and Caesarean birth.

*Hatha Yoga for Total Health* by Sue Luby, Prentice-Hall, Inc., Englewood Cliffs, New Jersey, 1977. Comprehensive coverage of the anatomy of correct movement in yoga postures. Photos include arrows designating movements of parts of the body in the poses.

*Light on Yoga* by B.K.S. Iyengar, Schocken Books, New York, revised edition, 1979. The definitive book on yoga and yoga philosophy. The standard textbook of yoga postures. Written by B.K.S. Iyengar, a master teacher and practitioner of yoga poses for over 50 years. Includes an excellent introduction to yoga, over 200 illustrated yoga poses and variations, hints and cautions, techniques, benefits of each pose, breathing control practices, and detailed courses of study.

*Runner's World Yoga Book* by Jean Couch, World Publications, Inc., Mountain View, California, 1979. Excellent step by step stretching and strengthening poses adapted for stiff, as well as flexible, students. Includes anatomical information and stresses the benefits of yoga for the athlete.

*Stretch and Relax* by Maxine Tobias and Mary Stewart, The Body Press, a division of HPBooks, Inc., Tucson, Arizona, 1985. Beautifully designed and photographed book emphasizing the benefits of stretching poses. Includes brief sections on stretching in pregnancy, positions for labor, and stretching after birth.

*Yoga, a Gem for Women* by Geeta S. Iyengar, Allied Publishers Private Limited, New Delhi, India, 1983. Comprehensive book on the theory and practice of yoga for women. This book combines Geeta's insights into the needs of women with the knowledge gained by years of working with her father, Mr. B.K.S. Iyengar. Includes an illustrated section on poses and breathing practices appropriate during pregnancy.

*Yoga and Pregnancy* by Sophy Hoare, Unwin Paperbacks, London, England, 1985. Indepth coverage of Iyengar yoga poses suitable during pregnancy. Clearly illustrated with photos and drawings. The author, an Iyengar yoga teacher and mother of four, has a thorough understanding of her subject and a warm, informative style of writing. Includes excellent information on the benefits of yoga, detailed pose descriptions, breathing and relaxation, changes during pregnancy, labor and birth, and correct poses after birth.

"Yoga and the Pregnant Woman", an article by Judith Lasater, Ph.D., R.P.T., *The IYTE Review*, Vol. 2, No. 1, a publication of the Iyengar Yoga Institute of San Francisco, California, 1981. A concise, highly informative article on the therapeutic benefits of yoga and relaxation during pregnancy and after birth. Covers the effects of pregnancy on the muscular, respiratory, cardiovascular, digestive, and nervous systems. Includes yoga poses for specific problems of pregnancy. Explains order of poses to be performed postpartum.

# Index

# Notes